BREAKABLE

ii

BREAKABLE

ॐ

Everything I know
about health,
and how it went wrong

SUE JULIANS

Published by New Generation Publishing in 2023

Copyright © Sue Julians 2023

First Edition

The author asserts the moral right under the Copyright, Designs and Patents Act 1988 to be identified as the author of this work.

All Rights reserved. No part of this publication may be reproduced, stored in a retrieval system or transmitted, in any form or by any means without the prior consent of the author, nor be otherwise circulated in any form of binding or cover other than that which it is published and without a similar condition being imposed on the subsequent purchaser.

ISBN: 978-1-80369-742-0

www.newgeneration-publishing.com

New Generation Publishing

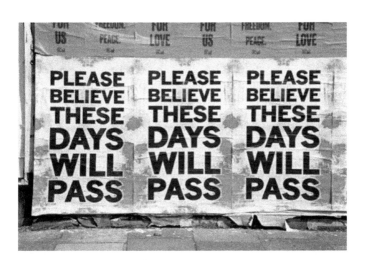

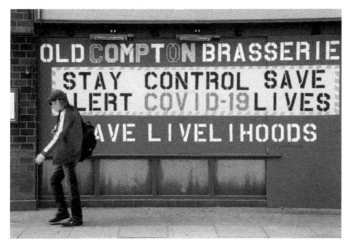

vi

Contents

Foreword xi

1 Bias and Priors 19

2 Prologue: My Rules for Living 24

3 Don't Worry, It's Not Covid 54

4 The Lockdown Battle for Business Survival 61

5 Reasons To Be Fearful: Part One 81

6 London in Lockdown 91

7 My Crash (and Burn) Course in Post-Viral Illness 105

8 The Kids Are (Not) All Right 116

9 The Great Unlock of London 126

10 The Adults Aren't All Right Either 137

11 Reasons To Be Fearful: Part Two – The New Normal . 144

12 The Circuit (Spirit) Breaker 153

13 'Tis the Season To Be 'Tiery' 156

14 The Bleak Midwinter 164

15 The Nightingale 172

16 Unintended Consequences 186

17 The Resistance To Reopening 194

18 School's Out Forever 199

19 British Summertime 207

20 What To Do, What To Do, What To Do? 211

21 A Very Different Capital City 216

22 Under the Bell Jar 223

23 Plan B: The 'Low-Cost' Cause of Long Covid? 231

24 Don't Worry, It *Is* Covid 237

25 Epilogue: My Rules for Life 242

26 Reconciliation 247

Appendix I – Coronavirus Restrictions Timeline............... 252

Acknowledgements 262

For

my husband and children

with love

x

Foreword

Future historians will probably struggle to deal with the mass of accounts of everyday life generated by the Covid-19 pandemic. The human experiences of past pandemics have vanished, where official records have survived. We must look for diaries, like those of Samuel Pepys recording middle-class reactions to the Great Plague of London in 1665; fallible memories, as in Defoe's *Journal of the Plague Year*, looking back on the same outbreak fifty years later; or imaginative reconstructions, like Connie Willis's *Doomsday Book*, where a time traveller encounters the Black Death, or Reina James's *The Time of Dying* – an undertaker's view of the 1918 influenza pandemic. Covid-19 has, however, been the first social media virus, with a plethora of tweets, posts and blogs documenting the fears, uncertainties and conflicts of a wide cross section of the populations of richer countries at least. Just as with any study of everyday life, other reactions are hard to capture in an enduring form: those of the poor, the socially marginal and the socially excluded, whether as groups within the Global North or as whole nations of the Global South.

Breakable, though, stands out from the crowd. Sue Julians, its author, is an acute observer of the impact of the restrictions imposed on the people of London by the policy and management choices adopted by UK politicians and public health leaders in response to the virus. Lockdown was never inevitable: it was a human decision made by those with the power to make it. But this account is also a reflective one. Sue Julians is an experienced physiotherapist, accustomed both to dealing with clients in pain and distress and to informing her work by critical evaluation of evidence. The book charts her growing disillusion with the management of the pandemic and the refusal of policy elites to accept the harms being inflicted by their policies. She is also sensitive to the waste of resources, particularly in her insider account of the Nightingale hospital, and the bureaucracy of recruitment to roles in call handling and vaccination.

The author is constantly aware of her privilege, as a well-off white woman living with her family in a nice residential part of the city. As her business in the Barbican twists and turns with each shift in policy, she and her children roam across the central city, noting the deserted streets and forlorn cafes. Occasionally, they witness or experience police harassment. If it was like this for me, she repeatedly asks, how bad was it for those less fortunate? How bad was it for those in overcrowded housing or living alone, without access to gardens and dependent on parks for open space and recreation, and required to use public transport daily to get to insecure jobs, servicing those who could comfortably work from home? Sue Julians is the canary in the coal mine, whose individual distress stands for the greater pressures and disruptions experienced by so many of her fellow Londoners.

The book is particularly moving in its account of the impact of pandemic restrictions on the lives of the author's children. They have been very brave to let her publish some of the details, but these are vital to aid our understanding of how indifferent many public health figures were to the consequences of their actions for those still in school or at university. The UK has a great tradition of public health work to improve or advocate for children's health and well-being. This has been a major driver of public health services for more than a century. Midwives, health visitors, school nurses and their medical equivalents have been at the forefront of campaigning for better health care, income support and protective services for children. All this was abruptly set aside. The damage to Sue Julians' children, their friends and all their contemporaries was dismissed as trivial, or a passing inconvenience from which they would bounce back because 'everybody knows' that 'children are resilient'.

This is a book that has contemporary resonance. Siren voices still call for public health restrictions every time there is an uptick in infection rates from respiratory viruses. Sue Julians adds her voice to those who insist that restrictions cannot be dismissed as bearing no costs or harms. There was never sufficient evidence of effectiveness to justify their duration and the use of state power to enforce them, and there was a reluctance to look for such evidence to replace simple, and simplistic, assertions by eminent scientists and medics. But it is also a book that should endure. When the next pandemic arrives, as it surely will, this volume should be on the library shelves, ready to warn policymakers against rolling over the playbook from Covid-19 and applying it to the next challenge.

Robert Dingwall

Nottingham, January 2023

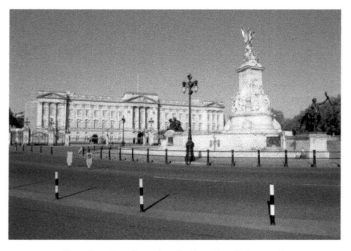

London landmarks during Lockdown 1

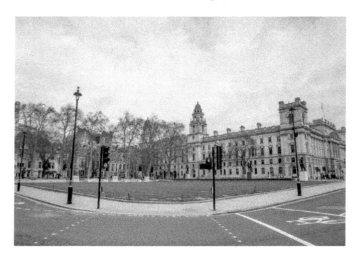

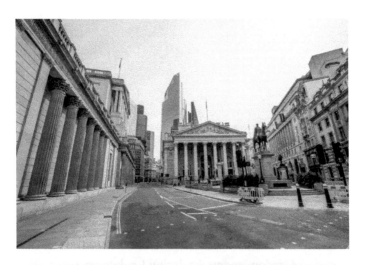

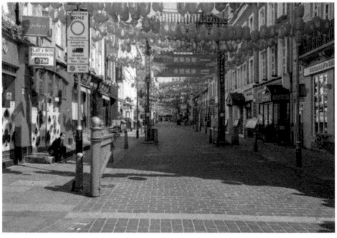

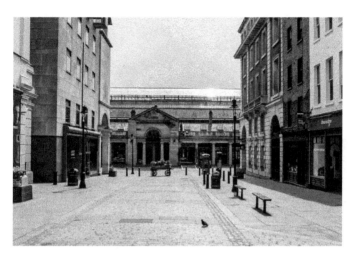

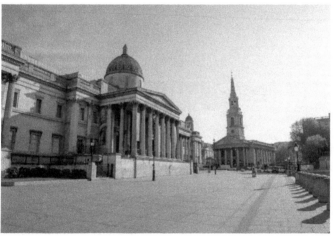

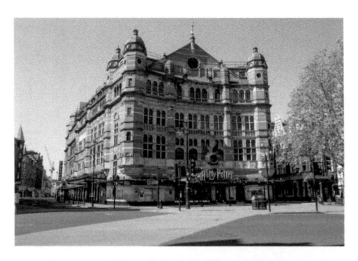

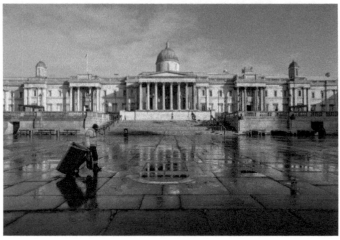

1 Bias and Priors

My career has been dedicated to improving quality of life. Through my training and my ongoing education at the hands of my patients, I have had the privilege of learning just how precious and fragile good health is. And how unique the cocktail of individual coping mechanisms required to maintain it.

Although it may be easy to consider our bodies as a collection of individual parts, we should not think of human beings as machines. We cannot simply switch ourselves on and off at will, expecting to function just as smoothly after a period of neglect.

Good health is effortful, not effortless, even when our healthy activities are so habitual that this effort is subconscious. Although we understand that taking exercise and eating well will benefit specific aspects of our health, we don't necessarily take the time to consider their knock-on effects on our well-being as a whole. But each system of our body relies on the others and cannot be considered in isolation.

The circumstances dictated by our ever-changing environment will determine the limits of our health and well-being. If our environment is conducive to health and all our systems are working well, our resulting quality of life and resilience to illness will be greater than the sum of these well-functioning parts. But the reverse is also true: if one part of the system is under pressure, all others will be adversely affected, and if our environmental coping mechanisms are taken away, the maintenance of good health may become an impossibility. This knowledge, together with my personal bias, became the lens through which I observed the pandemic unfolding.

Additionally, and unusually, I witnessed the effects of coronavirus restrictions in person. I treated patients face to face throughout, bar the two months between March and May 2020 when my professional body forbade it. I trained for Test and Trace and as a vaccinator. I worked at the Nightingale hospital in London in addition to working at my clinic. I have been exposed to other people's reality in their communities, observing and recording people's history, quality of life and all-round health because it is my professional responsibility to do so.

What I witnessed and experienced during the pandemic wasn't in the newspapers or on the television news. Looking at tables in bookshops groaning with coronavirus analyses, I see little representation of what life was like for me or the people I met.

Instead, this was a crisis calculated in graphs and predictions. The average human will make the average sacrifice to exert a similarly downward pull on the reproduction number of a virus. But we have lived through this crisis as individuals. There has been no average experience because there is no such thing as an average human. We lived our lives in parallel, not together. Our experiences, even if similar and familiar, were isolated from those of others.

I do not dispute the direct risks or harms of the pandemic. I know these would have been significant and devastating, regardless of the Public Health approach to managing it. My reason for writing this is to provide a different perspective: whilst the harms of Covid have been discussed at length, those of restrictions have not. There still seems to be an element of surprise and incomprehension at the range and extent of these harms, and I hope my book helps people to understand why some of them were a predictable and inevitable outcome of the policies chosen to attempt to control this virus.

Of course, we all have bias. I am a physiotherapist, a mother to school-aged children, a small-business owner and a city-centre resident. The risks of restrictions far outweighed those of an infection I had already suffered. But the full range of possible adverse effects caused by taking action wasn't modelled in advance, during, or it seems likely, in retrospect.

To my mind this is why personal histories are important: they tell the stories that would otherwise stay silent. They protest against the sweeping of this unrecorded, unmodelled damage under the carpet. They challenge the orthodoxy and the curation of a fiction that these harms either didn't happen or were unavoidable, and in doing so, they challenge the premise that lockdowns were successful when considered in the round.

What I have attempted to do is record what it was like to be in the thick of it. To witness our vibrant capital city as an apocalyptic ghost town. To tell the stories of those I met personally and professionally.

This is my story. My background, my history, my professional right to comment in this space. My reaction and interpretation as the pandemic unfolded. When I was wrong, and when I was, sadly, painfully right.

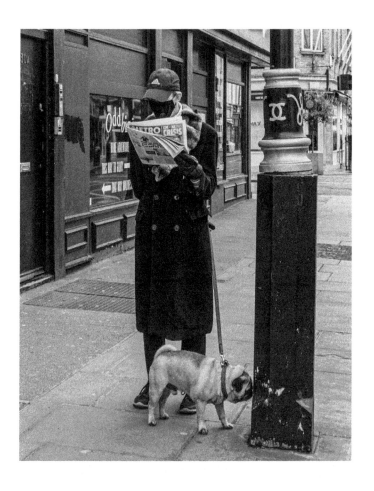

2 Prologue: My Rules for Living

In January 2020 I felt very lucky.

I had a happy and healthy family, a job I loved, a great work–life balance (most of the time), friends who were loyal and fun, and enough resources to enjoy my life to the full. I felt very calm and content. I was grateful for the times in my life when my plans had come to fruition, but I learned more from my failures than my successes. Had I achieved the accolades and credentials I aspired to, I would not have achieved the balance so personal to me and so essential to my well-being.

I attended the local state school and lived with my English parents and three older brothers; my family had moved to Scotland just before I was born. I don't remember a time when I didn't push myself to come first and do my best. Perhaps growing up with older brothers meant I had to push hard to be noticed or even to be considered their equal, given that I felt shoehorned into female stereotypes at the time.

I really wanted to become a doctor, but I was told by my local GP, my careers advisor and my own family that medicine was not a job for women. I was also advised against taking a degree in mathematics, physics or music due to concerns these wouldn't guarantee future employment. My parents had a point: in the early 1980s unemployment in the UK exceeded 10%. The television series *Boys from the Blackstuff*, a fictional account of unemployment in Thatcherite Britain, had put a bomb under the collective consciousness of my parents' generation; I remember my mother in particular was extremely upset by it. There would be a limit to the safety net my parents could provide. Although it was highly unlikely that I would share the fate of Yosser Hughes, who became increasingly desperate as the series went on, losing his children, his home and at one stage attempting suicide, they were understandably disinclined to support my creative or academic aspirations because of the risk that I might end up in an unfulfilling, insecure job. Or no job at all.

Instead, I was advised to undertake vocational training in something I would be able to do part-time after having children. My mum suggested following my grandfather's path. Having lost his leg at the Battle of Mons in the First World War, he was invalided out of the army and trained as a physiotherapist at the Royal Derby Hospital, running a private practice from his home until well into his seventies. Having decided that I wanted to work in a therapeutic role, and desperate to spread my wings, I left school at sixteen after my Highers. (Highers are the end-of-school exams. In Scotland these are a one-year course and count as three-fifths of an English A level. This difference explains why Scottish university degrees take four years rather than three.) I moved to London shortly after my seventeenth birthday to study at Guy's Hospital School of Physiotherapy.

I was woefully unprepared. My fellow students all seemed confident, gregarious and fitted in quickly. I was socially clumsy, naive, innocent and overwhelmed by both the hyper socialisation and debauchery of student life, as well as the sophistication and social confidence of my fellow students. I tried to project a persona of someone older and more worldly-wise but failed miserably.

I'd never tasted an olive or an avocado, never eaten an Indian takeaway. I didn't know how to play bridge or do the cryptic crossword. I was surrounded by accents I'd previously assumed were television parodies. Nobody could understand my Glaswegian accent, and since they spoke in a privately educated, middle-class language with constant references to a life I had no experience of, I struggled to understand them too. I had no filter, was direct to the point of rudeness, and found my contemporaries extremely difficult to read. I never felt I belonged, however hard I tried and however desperate I was to fit in.

It didn't help that physio students were fairly low in the college hierarchy: medics first, then dentists. Physios and radiographers were on a par below them. Nurses were at the bottom. This was my first experience of being thought of as somehow 'less' due to my sex, my class and my profession. Ironically, I now believe that being a physio is the best job within healthcare, at least for me. My mum was quite right to recommend it.

Physiotherapy aims to improve quality of life. Whether that's improving lung function, relearning and maintaining activity after a stroke, or treating a sprained ankle, we help patients overcome their difficulties to recover and maintain their physical function. It is extraordinarily rewarding, with considerably less risk of causing serious harm than in other healthcare professions. Our training is targeted towards the understanding of how our anatomy and physiology work together as an integrated whole, starting with the study of normal function, and then moving on to pathologies that disrupt our mind and bodily systems. Afterwards we study techniques to facilitate, maximise and maintain recovery to achieve optimal fitness and function. Within the physiotherapy school itself, we spent an extraordinary amount of time poking and prodding each other in our underwear. After learning how to identify bony parts, different muscles and normal ranges of movement, we learned the techniques of massage, manual therapy and exercise therapy to help relieve pain and improve function.

Some of our lectures took place in the medical school. I had the privilege of attending a guest lecture given by Sir Roger Bannister, the first man to run a mile in under four minutes. I remember thinking that he seemed such a nice, kind man with a benevolent manner. In a gentle voice he described the function of macrophages as the 'munch, munch, munch' clean-up mechanism of cells, and ever since then I've thought of them as teeny-weeny Pac-Men.

Dr Mike Hutchinson led our dissection lessons. Dr Hutchinson was responsible for many of the dissections featured in *Gray's Anatomy*, an essential medical textbook. Walking into his laboratory was an assault on the senses: the strong smell of formalin, coupled with the hundreds of pots on display containing different body parts floating in liquid made many students feel rather unwell. I remember looking up one day to be startled by a human spinal cord, dissected out as far as the nerves of the hands and feet, and displayed in an enormous square display case mounted on the ceiling. Much more of his work can be seen in the Gordon Museum – an anatomy museum that still exists within the grounds of Guy's Hospital. I was delighted to discover that, even now, he lectures occasionally at Guy's, some thirty-five years after he taught me and some fifty years since he started. He seemed brilliantly eccentric: whilst many of my peers were trying not to faint, he seemed as excited as a puppy each time he cut into a fresh cadaver.

After the first year our time was split between college and clinical placement: six weeks in, six weeks out.

One of my first placements was a general medical rotation including cardiac rehabilitation. During one ward round I was asked to take a man who had suffered a recent heart attack for a walk. Before doing this I checked his pulse, and his heart rate was 140 beats per minute. I reported this to the nurse in charge and told her I wasn't confident about his ability to walk without causing further harm. She told me I had to do it, that he needed to be discharged, and that he would either walk here or at home. Trusting her experience, I followed instructions. I walked with him around five metres from his bed, then five metres back. He promptly collapsed onto the bed, urinated, rolled his eyes back and died, right in front of my eyes.

Another placement – paediatrics – found me working in the neonatal intensive care unit and general paediatric ward: tiny, tiny babies, barely larger than my hand, incubated and intubated. My job was to expand and clear their lungs using the smallest suction tubes I had ever seen, similar in size to the straw you'd find taped to a can of WD-40, though much more flexible. The rest of my time was spent on the ward, mostly treating those with cystic fibrosis. There were two closely related families on that ward: one with nine children and one with thirteen. More than half these children had cystic fibrosis, and several of them had died before the age of twenty. The anger in one wee boy, who was thirteen years old and surely knew his fate, was unbearably tragic. It was no wonder he was reluctant to comply with the physio he found so difficult and painful.

After graduating in 1990 I took a rotational job as a junior physiotherapist at an NHS district hospital. Respiratory was my first rotation, combining intensive care with ward work. Our job was to clear patients' lungs of any obstruction restricting the flow of air and help those whose airways were less able to dilate and constrict. In intensive care this meant treating unconscious patients by inflating their lungs manually and using manual techniques to shake the chest and loosen lung secretions, before removing these with suction via their tracheostomy tubes. On the ward we would help people with chronic lung complaints. We inspected and tested the secretions that we helped them bring up from their lungs for colour, viscosity and smell so that we could help them improve their breathing and slowly, slowly their mobility.

My next rotation was care of the elderly. Here I learned how the maintenance of function relies on a co-dependent relationship between all systems of the mind and body. The ability of the elderly to recover from a specific illness may depend on any combination of a heart condition, lung condition, joint problem, confusion, metabolic illness and neurological complaint amongst others. I learned that, as life goes on, you steadily collect complaints, with death in the elderly, old or frail happening in stages over time as the body progressively shuts down, until it simply isn't strong enough to support life. It is possible, even inevitable, to die from old age if a serious single illness doesn't kill you first. It is also possible to delay this decline into frailty by socialising, eating a good diet and keeping both mind and body active. Not only do you improve your quality of life this way, but you also prolong it if you delay or slow down the process of frailty.

I enjoyed my next rotation in the stroke unit enormously. It was inspiring to learn neurological rehabilitation skills under the expert guidance of my senior physio, Lucy, who was a master in the application of the Bobath technique. This aims to reteach normal patterns of movement, avoiding the increase of muscle tone associated with primitive reflexes. I spent two hours a day for three months of this rotation working with one man, and I helped him relearn how to walk when he couldn't even sit unsupported at the start. Sadly, just before I finished the rotation, he had another massive stroke that he didn't survive.

I found my home in the musculoskeletal outpatients department. Jim and Roy, the two most senior clinicians in the department, were both completely blind. They were also two of the best clinicians I've ever had the privilege of working with. At that time blind physios were a regular part of the physiotherapy workforce, and they occupy an important part in the profession's history. (I also had three partially sighted lecturers during my training.) In 2019 the centenary of their participation in the profession was celebrated. Sadly, this seems to have steadily dwindled. The specially equipped North London School closed in 1995, and with the move of physiotherapy training away from hospitals, blind students were intended to be accommodated in universities instead. But far fewer are. With all the current emphasis on equality, diversity and inclusion, this feels like a bitter loss. I wonder how it was allowed to come about.

The musculoskeletal outpatients department, a large room with curtained cubicles, was navigated expertly by Jim and Roy without any aids: they knew exactly how many steps there were to the sinks and the cupboard, and woe betide any untidy junior who accidentally left something in the way.

A year into my junior job, a colleague asked if I would like to work for a local rugby union team in the evenings and at weekends. It was an easy way to see acute sports injuries (the NHS waiting list was a minimum six-week wait), so I eagerly joined her. A steep learning curve followed. I learned to strap ankles and wrists very, very speedily, and I quickly acclimatised to being surrounded by naked men, drinking beer and stinking of deep heat and sweat, in the changing rooms after each game.

During my fourth and final season, I ran onto the pitch having seen a player go down. He was clutching his knee. The players encircled him and were trying to reassure him when he screamed, 'It's not my fucking knee, it's my fucking shin!' Everyone's eyes dropped down simultaneously to see two obvious corners in his lower leg. The players turned away and slowly walked towards the changing room, whilst the manager ran to call for an ambulance. The attending GP was nowhere to be seen. The home side brought out the emergency kit.

Inside the bag I found an inflatable splint. One of the other players helped me take the injured player's boot off (no easy feat with a wobbly, unstable shin) and hold the leg whilst I gently guided the sleeve of plastic over it. The inflation tube was broken, but I managed to inflate it by lying in the mud to blow directly into the valve. The player was instantly more comfortable. When the ambulance finally arrived, I walked back to the changing room, longing for once for a cup of hot, sweet tea from the ubiquitous urn. Sadly, the lads had drained the pot and were sitting in stunned silence in the large communal bath, beers untouched.

Halfway through my time in rugby, I left my permanent job to work in a military hospital as a Senior Two, the next rung up on the career ladder. Patients here were predominantly military personnel with a smattering of local residents and inmates from Belmarsh prison. Wards were full of soldiers injured on duty or in conflict zones such as Northern Ireland, Bosnia and Rwanda. Some had the most horrific injuries. Working with these patients was humbling; they were very young men with missing limbs and eyes, ambushed or blown up by someone hiding out of sight with a remote trigger, poised to inflict maximum damage.

I heard many of these stories and found that the nature of their experiences did not match their demeanour, not one little bit. They were so calm and so matter-of-fact when relaying their appalling experiences.

I learned a lot about dealing with adversity, true adversity, in the two years I worked there, including what the patients needed to do to process it without breaking down. Some, of course, didn't manage this, especially those who joined up to escape an unhappy or abusive childhood. But those who were not broken by these most horrific of experiences were an inspiration. So, so calm. With a missing eye, a blown-off leg or widespread shrapnel injuries as a testament to a lifetime of physical pain and loss of function. So calm.

I dreaded to think of what horrors the soldiers had witnessed. And having spent my career learning how to improve people's lives and taking great personal reward from it, I also wondered at those who sat with their finger on a button, waiting for the perfect moment to maim or kill.

What also impressed me about these young men was how accepting they were of their fate. The camaraderie on the orthopaedic ward was inspiring: there was no sense of panic or anger, just a determination to recover. And a great deal of humour. These patients had been admitted for surgery and early-stage rehabilitation before being transferred to a high-level rehabilitation unit. We had the time and the facilities to see them several times a day. It was the most clinically rewarding job I have ever had.

The military hospital was also home to the regional burns unit. These patients were in a great deal of pain, and the physiotherapy for these injuries was very painful too. We had to stretch out their burned limbs, otherwise the scars from these burns would contract and render their joints useless and permanently frozen into bent, distorted shapes. Even worse, the healing of a circumferential burn could, if left alone, become a tourniquet cutting off all blood supply and resulting in gangrene and amputation. Physiotherapy was essential. On one occasion I was asked to see someone whose nether regions had been deliberately set on fire. He was a violent criminal, who had been chained to the bed, and he was less than pleased to have me stretch out his legs. After the first encounter I decided to hand this case over to one of my burly, male army colleagues.

I left my military and rugby positions in 1995 to study full-time for an MSc in neuromusculoskeletal physiotherapy at University College London. This was transformational for me as a clinician. Our first lecture, given by the extraordinary Ann Thomson, changed my practice forever. She stood at the front of the class and asked us whose approach to treatment we followed as clinicians. As each name was mentioned, she wrote it on the acetate of the overhead projector; it wasn't long before the projected image was full of names. The reason for asking the question was clear: with so many different approaches, not one of them had been found to work for all patients and all conditions. This was my introduction to clinical reasoning, the moving away from a recipe-style management towards one I could modify depending on the patient's characteristics and lifestyle.

The in-depth learning of different systems that I acquired during my MSc taught me how to decide on the right management for the individual, not just on their diagnosis. Studying the physiology of pain, control of movement and other homeostatic systems in depth helped me to understand why people respond so differently to interventions. I started to treat patients more holistically.

Many injuries will improve spontaneously with time and a simple approach. In the case of sprained ankles, most will simply heal with time, early rest and a gradual return to activity. Physiotherapy for this type of injury aims to ensure full recovery of strength, mobility and balance, and the prevention of recurrence. But a smaller proportion will not recover spontaneously. Often there are complaints with no obvious cause, for example, an office worker who develops neck and arm pain over several months with no history of trauma. Sometimes it's a patient with the most simple diagnosis who does not improve either spontaneously or by following a standard clinical pathway. To be successful with this cohort of trickier patients, you need to be committed to listening and learning from them all. If you only treat diagnoses by repeating previous treatments, your patient mileage will not improve your skills over time. (Patient mileage is the term used to describe the accumulation of clinical experience through individual cases.) You need to treat not only the condition but also the person who owns it.

My clinical reasoning had improved, but after transferring into the private sector post-Masters, there were new challenges to overcome. It isn't enough to have excellent skills in assessment and treatment, the patients also have to like you. My social skills had to improve, and fast. There would be no steady stream of guaranteed work. If patients were not comfortable with you, you didn't give them what they wanted, or you didn't get results, they would find someone else. To help establish a connection, I started reading the newspaper in its entirety, even the sports section, to have something to discuss. Small talk became easier.

What I hadn't predicted was the amount of clinically relevant information that came from the ensuing conversations. A casual chat about football would segue into their concerns for the child or ageing father they took with them to matches. One senior lawyer, when asked about her work, told me she had only had two hours of sleep since Monday – and this was Thursday. People talked about their lives, what was important to them, their aspirations and their fears. I learned that outward confidence commonly disguises an inner struggle. These successful individuals curated what they showed to the world, but underneath they had the same stresses and strains as everyone else.

I started to enjoy these chats. When patients came back with a different problem, I could remember the names of their children, where they'd been on holiday, if they had a sick relative or if they were due to move home. I realised that the differences between patients with the same conditions were not just their jobs, hobbies and bodies, they were mental differences too. And their combined relevance for prognosis and recovery started to become more obvious.

I find people fascinating. Not their environment so much, but how they respond to it, their coping strategies and what makes them tick. How differently they respond and their capacity for work, exercise and stress. How they manage, or don't manage, to override their body's needs through sheer force of will, and what happens when this ability is lost. I studied CBT (cognitive behavioural therapy) and anxiety, and I delved deeper into the effects of stress, powerlessness at work and other factors impacting chronic illnesses. Eventually, this became my niche area of practice; my awareness of these effects meant that I could tailor my interventions more successfully.

My first job in private practice was nothing if not diverse. The company I worked for had contracts with fourteen different musical theatre productions and was well known throughout show business, sport and politics. It was a little intimidating but never dull. On one memorable morning I stepped out of my treatment room at 8 am to find a Secretary of State, a member of the England football team and a West End performer waiting in reception for their appointments. The performer had arrived in his pyjamas and dressing gown; as he stood up sleepily and rubbed his eyes, he explained, unnecessarily, that he wasn't really a morning person and apologised for his appearance. Much to my amusement he had not noticed or didn't know the identity of the other occupants of our tiny reception area.

Having treated one of Disney's senior executives, I became the primary physio looking after their new show, *The Lion*

King. This was the show I knew better than any other: I sat through many rehearsals to familiarise myself with the unique challenges it would present – there is even a moment where I filled the frame in the BBC *Panorama* special. Would the bungees that attached the giraffe heads to the rest of their costumes be secure? Did all those on stilts have adequate treads underneath their crutches?

It helped that I have always loved theatre. On several occasions I had already seen the production before one of the stars attended for treatment. For example, I knew that one actor presenting with neck pain was spending an hour of each performance sitting on a sofa with her head turned to the left in *Who's Afraid of Virginia Woolf?* – for eight shows a week.

It was a challenge to give these performers what they needed in addition to what they wanted. They would be seeking a passive treatment, a manipulation 'click' to help them feel temporarily better, and they were often not interested in addressing the underlying reason for their complaint. I found it difficult to motivate them to do enough remedial exercises to compensate for the asymmetrical nature of the choreography they were performing for eight shows every week. A dancer may only kick with one leg during the entirety of their performance, so exercise is important to maintain physical balance and avoid the development of overuse problems.

On one occasion I was sent backstage to treat a Shakespearian actor before the performance. This patient's lead role required him to die by falling backwards at the end of the play, and he didn't have enough strength or flexibility to perform this without losing control and causing low back pain through the compression of his lumbar spinal joints. I suggested that he attempt to fall with control, by using a little abdominal contraction to act as a braking mechanism. But he looked at me blankly before asking me for a massage and telling me he would like to sleep whilst this treatment was administered.

On another occasion when attending a star of a different West End show, I turned up with the company's portable treatment couch, only to find it was broken and unusable when I unfolded it. The actor was extremely frustrated and angry with me for not being able to 'click' her spine in the way she wanted pre-performance. I had seen this show and greatly admired this actor, who was Scottish, like me, and I managed to make her painful movements pain-free by treating her back slightly differently from the way she wanted. But she sent me away with a flea in my ear, and I wasn't asked to go back.

Though I really enjoyed working with these patients, it was very hard work. It was normal to see eighteen patients a day for half an hour each, and we were expected to work regular Saturdays too. Nine hours of clinical work may not sound much, but physio is very draining, both physically and mentally. And, as in the rugby environment, there was considerable pressure to pass the performers fit when they were not, both from the performers themselves and the company managers. I treated many famous actors, even some Hollywood movie stars. But I found it even more difficult to maintain my clinical objectivity when faced with a household name.

In 2000 I moved to a practice in the City of London and started working with companies and office workers, mainly in law and finance. They were no less interesting than my performers at the Harley Street practice, at least to me. Perhaps this was because I had more in common with them. They were also easier to reason with: they were more likely to take my advice on rehabilitation and prevention of future injury. Or, if they hadn't taken this advice the first time they attended with a non-traumatic injury, they would accept it on the second or third visit. I've lost count of the number of times my patients stopped exercising as soon as their pain settled, only to repeat the same behaviours that caused their painful complaint in the first place.

Musculoskeletal physiotherapy patients can be split roughly into two distinct groups: patients who have disturbed function due to too much movement or load and those who developed a problem because they didn't move enough. Although I enjoyed meeting everyone, I found sports injuries less interesting to treat, largely because these office-worker 'weekend warriors' did not usually need expert input. Elite sport and performance are much more expert fields, but this was not the cohort I was working with. I found the tricky spinal complaints much more rewarding to treat, since, without the spontaneous tissue healing following an acute sports injury, I felt more responsible for their improvement.

The office patients worked long hours with tight deadlines and a great deal of emotional stress. I had to adapt the way I approached this group by figuring out ways for them to maintain their workload whilst having their movement goals built into their time at work when possible. I had to think unconventionally: asking someone to exercise regularly when they work from 9 am until 10 pm was quite a challenge.

I loved this job, but after I'd been there for two years, the owner sold it to the GP practice we shared the premises with. The GP practice was, in turn, in the process of selling it to a much larger corporate entity. Where I had previously enjoyed a lot of freedom and autonomy, the new bosses wanted me to sign a contract with completely different terms and conditions. I decided to set up on my own instead and became self-employed at the beginning of 2003.

To find out which location would be more popular, I rented rooms on both Harley Street and Old Street for two days a week. After a year I worked solely in the busier Old Street practice and recruited my first employee. In 2004 I sold my flat to finance a move into premises of my own and secured my first corporate contract with a large firm of solicitors.

Having managed to weather the global financial crisis of 2008, I secured another corporate contract in 2012.

Unfortunately, my landlord decided to sell the building and told me that my lease would not be renewed. There followed a mad scramble to find alternative premises. At one point I considered buying premises to avoid a repeat of my prohibitive service charges, my repairing and renewal lease, and the risk of my lease not being renewed. However, the difficulty of finding anything with the right use was challenging. Medical clinics, along with educational institutions, are listed as D1 properties by local councils, and physios can only practice from premises with this usage classification. At one point I had progressed sufficiently in the purchase of premises on City Road to the point of changing my pension into one that could be used towards the purchase of a commercial property. The estate agent assured me he had seen the paperwork confirming this property had D1 use. Unfortunately, it did not. A planning application to convert it to D1 was subsequently refused, and I had to pull out of the purchase.

Eventually, I was approached by someone who wanted to sell their practice and retire. After a drawn-out process, more stressful than anticipated, I set up a limited company and acquired Barbican Physio, combining both businesses and moving there in January 2015. Between then and January 2020 gross turnover increased by 240%, and we had become a team of six physiotherapists, two admin staff and numerous other professionals who rented space from me. I'd added a third corporate contract and was responsible for providing physio services to any of the 8,000 staff members who wanted to access treatment at work.

☙

I married in 2005 and had my first child two years later. Two weeks overdue, I had a dreadful labour for two days, including twelve hours on a syntocinon drip (which gave me three uterine contractions every ten minutes) with no pain relief. The epidural hadn't worked. Even after that, my cervix was still only one centimetre dilated, and I ended up with an emergency Caesarean section. Still exhausted and struggling to feed my wakeful, hungry newborn, I returned to work two weeks later when my landlord issued an enormous bill for changes to the building following the Disability Act. All these costs were to be met by leaseholders, with my share being £10,000.

Four months later I had pneumonia. Nine months after my baby was born, I broke down completely when an absolutely hideous image came into my head. I imagined putting a knife to my chest and ending it all. My heart was racing. No matter how deeply I breathed, how much I tried to calm myself and use the CBT training I'd had, nothing made a difference. I didn't know if I needed to call 999. To find out if I did, I went to the kitchen and put a knife to my chest to see if I really wanted to do it. But I didn't. I put the knife away and tried to sleep. Every two hours I was woken by the same racing heart – twenty minutes up and twenty minutes down. I learned to simply wait for it to pass.

I saw my GP the next day. I had seen her recently for something routine, and she had told me then that she was worried I was sliding into postnatal depression. It was clear she was right, though I protested it at the time. She put me on antidepressants. Although the panic attacks worsened for the next two to three days, they then stopped, and I haven't had them since. It took me much longer to feel any emotion, but at least I could function.

When I became pregnant for the second time, I started to feel scared it would happen again. My GP referred me to a private obstetrician, to whom I recounted my terrible labour and the aftermath. We planned an elective Caesarean section, and she referred me to a psychiatrist.

When I spoke about my life to this wonderful woman, she asked me a simple question, 'But who looks after you, my dear?' I sat open-mouthed. 'You're not superwoman,' she said. She told me how the images in my head had been put there by my body to force me to take notice and slow down. They had become more and more awful until I finally gave in and asked for help. She advised me to resume taking the antidepressants because it was better for the baby that I was calm rather than riven by stress.

When I saw her again three weeks later, she said immediately, 'Ah! You're better! I was pretty sure it was state, not trait.' I asked her to explain. She told me that I had clearly been acutely mentally unwell but that this wasn't part of my normal personality. She warned me that I would risk a relapse if I were to undergo another period of prolonged stress. I resolved to look after myself a little better.

At her recommendation I saw a psychologist to make sure I wasn't developing behaviours that would limit or prevent my recovery. She told me I was doing almost everything she would have recommended, but she had two pieces of advice for me. One: don't avoid knives; force yourself to use them and break the catastrophisation trigger entirely. Two: try to find something positive to take away from this experience.

This made me quite cross. How could anything good come from this? My confidence had gone. I had been through the worst experience of my life and thought I would never recover, not completely. But over time I realised that she was right. I had learned empathy. I understood properly what it felt like to be vulnerable and powerless. This humbled me; I had new insight into myself and those around me.

I also gained an understanding of mental illness. I had been acutely unwell, but it was not my fault. Once I became unwell, changing my behaviour wasn't enough to overcome it. I could not control my heart rate by breathing deeply, and I could not stop myself from waking up with a racing heart in the middle of the night. I was grateful that for me, at least, this illness was temporary and recoverable.

I began to recognise vulnerability in others. I saw that people's unexpected behaviour is often not personal; it belies an inner struggle. So, take a deep breath, don't take offence, and give them the benefit of the doubt rather than respond in a retaliatory manner.

ଔ

I approached parenthood like I approach most other areas of my life: by trying to be as well informed as possible. I had already learned about physical development and milestones during my physiotherapy training. And as part of our psychology module, I learned about critical periods of psychosocial development. These occur at different stages of childhood when neurological pathways increase at an enormous rate. If milestones are not met within those times, they may not be met at all. I learned that this explosion of white matter also accounted for toddler tantrums and teenage emotional distress, when this sudden increase of emotion would leave these children frustrated and confused. The distress would continue until the pathways settled through both repeated environmental exposure to their established behaviours and the reinforcement of expected outcomes. They are critical periods for this reason: if you don't develop certain abilities within these periods, you may not develop them at all. Worse, you may develop pathways that can continue to adversely affect your health and happiness throughout your life.

During my pregnancy I read everything I could. One email newsletter charted the course of my baby's growth from a peanut to a watermelon. Out of professional curiosity I read extensively about physical changes and how to manage or prevent pain and loss of function. Having educated myself and attended a few health courses on physiotherapy for pregnant women, I became rather angry about the way women were treated through pregnancy. One of my friends referred to it as 'being treated as a second-class citizen within your own body'. It did irk me somewhat to be asked, 'How is baby?' at the start of every midwife appointment.

Many physical complications of pregnancy can be prevented or lessened. I had two enormous babies but didn't have a diastasis recti (splitting of the abdominal muscle). I did not suffer for long from pelvic girdle pain because I knew which behaviour I needed to change to try to stop it, or at least prevent it from becoming debilitating. But this advice was absent from my antenatal care. Even as an 'elderly primigravida' at the grand old age of thirty-seven, it felt like I was treated as no more than a vessel for the baby.

I read a wide range of books on how to look after my baby, everything from Gina Ford's works to *The Baby Whisperer* on sleep, and from strict feeding times and amounts to baby-led weaning. As soon as my children appeared, I realised these opinions and books were just like the various approaches to treatment I had learned as a clinician. Not one approach suits every baby or every mother. Or, as a friend told me, 'The problem is, the baby hasn't read the books.'

The clear differences between children, even newborns, surprised me. I'd thought of children as being largely blank canvases. Of course, they would look like their parents and perhaps have the same talents or lack thereof, but I had assumed their personalities were more likely to be dictated by their upbringing rather than their genetic inheritances. But it soon became clear that their personalities were a product of both nurture and nature: not only in the way they behaved socially, but also in what activities would soothe them and give them their quality of life. I made it my ambition as a parent to find out what these were, hoping that by the time my children left home they would be not only independent, well educated and able to form strong relationships, but also aware of what they would need to be able to relax and find their work–life balance.

ಬ

As a physio it is my job to help patients recover, and to educate and empower by giving them control of their health. Sometimes the challenge is to find what the patient has the power to change, expanding your focus, rather than adopting a prescriptive response to a specific injury or condition.

We need both exercise and relaxation to maintain mind and bodily health. Our autonomic nervous system gears us up for activity by increasing our blood pressure and the blood supply to our muscles. But we also need to relax to allow our body time to repair itself, digest our food and prepare for the next burst of activity. Imbalance in this stress–relax cycle will, at some point, lead to ill health.

Our capacity for mental and physical stress is very individual. Some people can work harder and longer than others. But everyone has a threshold, and if you go beyond it, you will become unwell. I sometimes wonder if those who are commonly unwell during their holidays have unwittingly pushed themselves beyond the threshold just before it, and the drop in circulating stress hormones due to finishing work has allowed their body to produce symptoms forcing them to slow down and let their body repair. To relax mentally, some need a competitive stimulus, something to distract them from their life stressors. Like banging your elbow then rubbing it: the mechanical stimulus of the rubbing travels faster than the pain, blocking the signal. Mindfulness and meditation may only expose these patients to their inner cognitive fidget, sometimes giving them a feeling of panic or occasionally feeding their narcissism. They relax through competitive sports, CrossFit or strength and conditioning work, or by socialising or watching a movie.

Some people are less reliant on external influences or competitive goals for their relaxation. Their drive is internal, meditative and perhaps more on the creative side. Because they like to feel in tune with their bodies, they are drawn to exercise like yoga, running or swimming. To relax they may enjoy cooking, playing the piano, creating art or DIY. They benefit from feeling their bodily systems work synchronously, getting into a 'zone' of perfect balance as their mind and body work together, or by creating something they feel proud of.

In my experience you need to pick the exercise to match your patient's psychological profile to have any chance of ensuring they will continue it after their symptoms have settled. Staying out of pain becomes a positive side effect of the activities they continue for reasons of mental health and work–life balance. As it is my job to help them try to achieve the former, it is also my job to discern the latter.

I often think about these commonly found variations in character between the shy and the confident, between those inclined to creativity and those inclined to measurable, competitive goals: the yoga lovers and the CrossFitters. As I learn more from observing how my children and other children learn to navigate life, accumulating their layers of protection and resilience, I imagine the unconditioned, naive children hidden within the adults I interact with, and how these inherent characteristics and pathways of experience emerge at times of stress and unhappiness when the layers of armour and coping mechanisms are stripped away.

My teenage idea of success had been based on academic achievement, credentials and status. But as time went by, the more I realised that for me, these were false gods. I have met many people with glittering careers who are unfulfilled, unhappy in their relationships and permanently anxious. As a younger adult this puzzled me. These people had achieved the status and position in society I craved. But the only thing they knew how to do was to keep running and aim for the next target. They never learned when to stop and be happy with their accomplishments. They will never reach the pot of gold at the end of the rainbow.

I started to envy those who didn't need to satisfy their inner critic or seek the approval of others. Some don't need to have the best of everything or to constantly seek out the new and exciting. They work to live, demanding a work–life balance that the driven find so hard to achieve. Or perhaps they love the work they do so much that money and status are simply not a priority.

By January 2020 I had learned to allow myself to relax and find some contentment. The business was a success. I had paid off the previous owner six months before, and I had saved six months' rent and rates for a rainy day. I could start saving for a pension and would, for the first time, earn more than my best-paid employee. I had a busy but manageable life with just enough stimulus to keep me busy, but not so much that I couldn't relax. I had silenced my inner critic.

I felt very lucky.

3 Don't Worry, It's Not Covid

I am hypermobile. This means that the elastic-band quality of my connective tissues is much looser than that of others, giving increased flexibility and less stiffness. My scaffolding, made of rubber rather than steel, is less able to keep me upright without physical effort. That means I have to physically work harder: I walk on sand, where others walk on pavement. It makes physical activity more tiring, as I rely more than others on muscle strength and endurance rather than joint stiffness and elastic rebound for basic function. This lack of tension in my tissues also provides less feedback into neuromuscular coordination systems, and as a result, I am clumsy and have poor balance.

But once I work hard at learning a skill, I'm good at it. My coordination is excellent, possibly more so because of the need to overcome my hypermobility. I'm very good at parking cars or manipulating body parts. But I hate taking part in any activity with a high risk of injury. I sometimes joke that this is due to my job and the injuries I have seen, but the truth is that I cannot gauge my speed or that of others, and if tasked to make a quick physical calculation, I often make a mistake. Owing to my hypermobility, I have to be primed for physical action by the feed-forward predictability of it, and the unexpected will cause me to stumble or fall. When there is acute danger or a sudden change, I tend to freeze rather than act. (Feed forward describes the mechanism by which an outcome can be predicted by past experience, for example, the repeated practice of a tennis serve. Consciously, you may consider what type of shot you want to play, but your unconscious competence, derived from practice and repetition, determines the skill in performing the action.)

I have wondered if this is what led me to work increasingly with persistent conditions rather than with the sports and performance injuries of my early career. In the end sport left me cold. I couldn't understand why someone would risk wrecking their body to make every single performance or to play in every single match. I better understood those who felt an obligation regarding their office jobs or deadlines, perhaps because I, too, was able to work hard and long, and because I knew the difficulties in mentally overriding your body's capabilities in such a sustained and persistent manner.

I also wonder if this is why I now try to assess situations, all situations, on what might go wrong before I act. Why might this be wrong? What will be the unintended consequences? As an optimist I'm aware that I have sometimes made a bad decision if pressed to make it quickly. So, over the years I have tried to learn from my mistakes and be as cautious mentally as I am physically.

I was lucky enough to learn how to ski as a child on the slopes of Glenshee and Aviemore, and as an adult, my more privileged life allowed this to continue on the slopes of Europe. Although I'm clumsy and not very good, I've always loved skiing: the dreamless sleep enabled by clear, clean mountain air, the camaraderie of skiing with a group of friends and feeling the air rush by your ears whilst your skis glide over cotton-wool snow. Being able to eat and drink what you like and wake up without a headache is also an enormous benefit: every country seems to have a unique libation best enjoyed to excess.

It also reminds me of my dad, who died six weeks after my second child was born. At his funeral, my brother's eulogy included the familiar tale of 5 am rises, three jumpers, home-made skis and four-hour drives to Glenshee. My dad would park where it was free, half a mile from the lifts: I still remember those long walks in ill-fitting boots. We would return home late at night with twelve pence left, having had just enough cash to buy us a fish supper from the chippie in Auchterarder on the way home.

My dad was a man of few words but many eccentricities. He was an engineer by trade (having trained through an apprenticeship at Rolls-Royce) and when he died, the inventory from his garage included seventeen broken strip lights, bags of corks and boxes stuffed full of little bits of wire. Every screw had been meticulously catalogued, labelled, kept in old jam jars and stored on home-made shelving with perfectly crafted slots for each jar to slide into. I adored him.

As an adult I joined him for several skiing trips with his old work colleagues. I have a cherished photo of the moment his magnificent eyebrows froze into antlers after skiing through the clouds in Tignes. Later that day he joined me and my new boyfriend (now my husband) in our hotel for the seafood buffet night. What a joy it was to watch him feast his eyes and then his belly on the cornucopia of delights that awaited.

When faced with delicious food he would manage a series of appreciative moans and sighs, with the occasional punctuation of 'magnificent', or 'ooh, that is just the essence of blackcurrant' in his untamed Derbyshire accent.

Skiing felt like being closer to him: his love of food, companionship and the skiing itself. And he was a beautiful skier. Long, slim skis (before the era of carvers), knees and ankles almost touching, as he elegantly, slowly threaded his way down even the deadliest black. It was a joy to watch.

St Anton was his favourite resort. Although we hadn't been there with him, after his death my brother and I planned a trip with our families. 2020 was the fourth or fifth time we had been there together, hoping to pass on this love to our children but always having a toast 'to Dad' during our trip.

This 2020 trip wasn't so enjoyable. On Wednesday 19 February, I woke with a sore back, which deteriorated through the morning. I booked a massage, thinking I had overdone it or carried my skis awkwardly. I was treated by an Australian physiotherapist, who was planning to move to London after the skiing season. I have often wondered what happened to her.

The massage didn't help my back, despite being expertly given. By lunchtime my whole spine was aching. After a two-hour nap my throat felt as if I'd swallowed ground glass; it was so, so painful. And I was incredibly tired; I found it difficult to leave my bed at all, only doing so to buy food or medication or to pick up the children from ski school. But it felt like I was wearing a suit of lead; my body was so heavy.

I called the local medical centre for advice. 'Not Covid,' they said, 'You have no temperature.' (At this stage the guideline for diagnostic purposes was a high temperature and a new, persistent cough.) I went back to bed. Two days later I struggled out to the pharmacy. I was reassured again. 'It's not Covid; it's safe to get on your flight home.' On the last night of the trip, my family persuaded me to go out to a restaurant with them. And I did. Drugged up to the eyeballs and feeling dreadful, but I did.

It turned out that I and many thousands of half-term skiers brought Covid to the UK from the Alps at the end of that week. Ischgl, only ten kilometres from us in St Anton, had been one of the hotspots for transmission. Despite being an exercise undertaken outside, it's no surprise to me that skiing was such a good environment for transmission. The close contact of skiers regularly throughout the day, whilst breathing heavily from altitude and exercise, was the perfect scenario to aid transmission.

Of course, none of us were tested. I knew a lot of people who had a nasty illness at that time, but they put it down to flu or a Gok (God only knows), as my late father-in-law, a paediatrician, would have described it. Not everyone had both symptoms of a persistent cough and a high temperature. Not everyone had access to an antibody test, unlike me. The antibody test I took in late May 2020 showed it had, in fact, been Covid all along.

From every part of the UK, people travelled by train or plane to the mountains of Europe. We converged cheek by jowl with a multiplicity of strangers in lift queues (with sniffle stops dispensing tissues), gondolas, chair lifts, transfer buses, lunch queues and bars. For those who don't ski, it's perhaps difficult to comprehend how close and repeated these contacts are: I find it difficult to imagine a day of skiing with fewer than one hundred close contacts. Because of this, I found it hard to believe those who subsequently claimed that locking down on 16 March rather than 23 March would have made a great deal of difference. I was more inclined to believe it was much more widespread and much earlier than was generally understood.

It took me a very long time to feel well again. The initial flu-like symptoms lasted for ten days and my persistent cough for six weeks. By then I was dealing with the prospect of lockdown and trying to stop my business from folding, so it's no surprise that this initial illness segued into something much longer lasting. I couldn't rest; I didn't have the choice.

At least once I knew I'd had Covid, survived it and exposed my entire family to it, we were less afraid of it. But this was a very thin silver lining on the huge series of dark clouds that were to follow.

4 The Lockdown Battle for Business Survival

March 2020 began twelve days after my first symptoms of Covid. I was just getting over the severe, acute fatigue, still coughing, and still sleeping twelve hours out of twenty-four. That luxury ended when February did: it felt like someone had plugged me into the mains or dumped me into a big glass cube and started filling it up with water.

Businesses had started to plan for remote working. I received a huge volume of emails from anxious staff, patients and companies. People were adrenaline fuelled, working all hours, scared and trying to get their heads around what it all meant. Many thought they would lose their jobs. A mad scramble followed for office equipment and adequate internet connections to run video conferencing from home.

How could we help our patients if they were stuck at home? What would the obvious, predictable problems be? We started to look at how to make Skype consultations work effectively (Zoom was yet to appear, at least in my consciousness) whilst remaining within our scope and rules of practice. I sought advice from my professional body, campaigned for remote consultations to be covered by health insurers, and started pleading with the landlord, the local council and the sources of our other fixed costs. I began to post on Twitter, looked carefully at my many insurances and even had a letter published in *The Times*.

People started panic buying essential goods. Images of empty shelves started gracing social media, particularly those usually stocked with toilet rolls and cleaning products. Small bottles of hand sanitiser started to sell for ludicrous sums: the only bottle I saw in the local pharmacy had a price tag of £80. Pasta, bread flour and yeast were also in very short supply. The contrast between the aisles of untouched fresh produce and those usually stocked with store cupboard essentials was striking. Queues started to form round the block at all food stores, with aisles holding non-essential goods taped off completely.

I was in denial. I'd lived through the BSE (bovine spongiform encephalopathy) crisis when harms turned out to be a small fraction of the prediction. I'd heard of swine flu, SARS (severe acute respiratory syndrome) and Ebola, all of which had died out before reaching the UK, or shortly afterwards. I hoped Covid would be the same, not least because I was sure that lockdown would cause serious harm, in addition to being disastrous for my business and the livelihoods of those who worked within it.

From the perspective of a physio, lockdown is the very opposite of what we advise patients to do; we advise them to stay physically active, separate work life from home life, maintain downtime and turn off devices regularly. We advise physically and mentally frail people to keep up their strength, fitness, mobility and interaction with others to slow their rate of decline and lead a longer and fuller life. Imagining the fallout from the policies being discussed was sobering. I knew people would not simply bounce back and the longer this went on, the worse it would be.

I had six months' rent and rates in a reserve account. This amount would cover my staff costs for only six weeks. I told my employed staff that I'd have to put them on half hours and half pay, hoping that within three months either I would have organised a loan or the office workers would have returned. My quote for a commercial loan was at 13% annual interest, terrifyingly unaffordable, particularly given that I had no idea how long it would be before my business could return to normal. So, I took the risk, refused the commercial loan, and hoped the office workers would soon be back. At this point neither the CBILS (Coronavirus Business Interruption Loan Scheme) nor furlough had been announced.

One of the worst experiences I had in this dreadful, dreadful month was telling my staff I didn't know how long I could pay them. All had families relying on my business to pay their mortgages and put food on the table. To have to communicate this news was simply one of the most distressing experiences of my life.

My fight with medical insurers was prolonged, and it sickened me. I had a constant feeling of nausea that threatened to rise up each time I knew I had to behave assertively on a call. Each time I picked up the phone or logged into Zoom, it felt like the outcome could mean the end of my business and the jobs it supported, and I had no power. We were a close-knit team and had worked together for years: the responsibility for this, always tricky, became a crushing and intolerable load.

In order to cover fixed staff and premises costs, I had calculated that we needed to conduct one hundred and five appointments per week. During the first week of March, we conducted one hundred and ninety-five physiotherapy appointments. In the second week this had dropped to one hundred and sixty-five. By the third week most companies had shut their offices and this number had dropped to fifty-four: a loss of around £3,000 for the week. By Friday 20 March only two medical insurers, covering less than 5% of our business, had agreed to cover virtual consultations. It was desperate. And the lockdown hadn't even started yet.

On 19 March I was in and out of virtual meetings all day with frantic side chats and requests for legal advice. I had to break off in the early evening to rush over to the Chelsea and Westminster Hospital for a hysteroscopy, an uncomfortable, invasive procedure. The clinic reception area was empty of patients, and I was last on the list. Tapping my foot, impatient to get on and get back to work, I had a very lively conversation with the consultant gynaecologist and his colleague before the procedure, (the poor man had asked if Covid had started to affect my business yet). The procedure itself was painful and undignified, but I confess I barely noticed it, bar the few yelps of pain I heard emanating from my own throat.

My mood afterwards was not improved when, by quickly checking my emails before getting dressed, I found out that my largest insurer had gone back on their word completely and would not, after all, be covering video consults with my practice, even though I had a contract with the companies to provide physio services to their staff. I'm not at all embarrassed to admit that I sank down on the hospital chair and wept for a few minutes before pulling myself together, wiping my cheeks with a sleeve, getting dressed and making my way back home. There I worked until midnight, restarted at 2 am and worked through until midnight came around again.

As a small independent I had very little to bargain with, so I had to play dirty to survive. If I hadn't succeeded, the separate legal entity of my limited company would not prevent my landlord from having a claim on my personal assets. I looked at putting my business into administration, cutting the cord and minimising my losses. But after a long conversation with my accountant, I realised this was not as simple as I had believed.

Like many limited companies, I pay myself a fixed salary of around half the national minimum wage as an employee, but I take most of my income in dividends. This allows for fluctuations in costs and income to be absorbed: in better months I take out a good amount, in other months, for example, when I pay my quarterly rent, I take out nothing.

During the first week of lockdown beginning on 23 March, we conducted twenty-three physiotherapy appointments, all online. A loss of £5,000. I had no government grant or help with business rates. Had I been a beautician, I would have received £50,000 in grants and rates relief, but I was in the wrong sector. It wasn't the chief medical officer who told us to close, it was our professional body. For that reason, we didn't qualify for government help. And as I worked through a limited company, I had no support for my income either.

Time seemed to simultaneously stand still and accelerate. After four hours of adrenaline-ridden, rapid-fire multitasking, my brain would freeze. I wouldn't know what to do next. I would start at pace with a list of things I could try to do, but after a while I hit the wall, and nothing worked. I couldn't think or see clearly what I needed to do next. And that's when the panic would start.

That was my cue to stop and go outside. When I lacked the insight to know I'd reached this point, my husband would find me staring into space and would drag me out to try to clear my head. Some of my friends had decided not to leave their homes at all, even for their permitted exercise. They had their food delivered, avoiding fresh foods (because they required refrigeration) and leaving everything in their hallway for three days before touching it. They didn't handle their post for three days either – and even when they did, they used disposable gloves to do so, carefully disposing of both the gloves and the wrapping after opening.

I lost all the colour in my life, all sharpness and meaning. I was sleepwalking fast with only the tinnitus of static interference, like the hissing and sputtering of an old black-and-white television, to accompany me. It felt like I was being plugged in repeatedly until a fuse blew. Go, stop, go, stop, go, stop. All other aspects of life were blocked out completely; I had no bandwidth for them. I felt nothing but intermittent surges of adrenaline, causing nausea and an increased heart rate to push me through the next task.

I was lucky, of course, with a happy house and a privileged life. I had a lot in the tank compared with others. I could, and would, get through. But I was completely numb, totally spent, emotionally switched off and wading through mud, one painful step at a time.

When lockdown was finally announced, there was an inevitability to it. We had all heard of the unfolding disaster in Italy and seen the images: bodies dying in corridors with hospitals completely overwhelmed. The Cheltenham Festival from 10 March to 13 March created a huge uproar. The images of thronging crowds, as large as 25,000, mixing without caution were juxtaposed with those images from Italy, and they made our government appear reckless and murderous.

Lockdown was sold to the public as a brief incarceration followed by a kind of 'get-out-of-jail/pandemic-free' card. We would 'squash the sombrero', making case numbers manageable and then slowly unwind restrictions, using test, trace and isolate to keep them at a low, controllable level. This would supposedly be enough to keep the dreaded R reproduction number under one, just as Asian countries had done with previous infectious diseases, particularly SARS, which was another coronavirus. (The reproduction number denoted how many future infections would be generated from each infection. Over one, the number of infections would be increasing; under one, they would be reducing.) We were encouraged to look to Asia for inspiration, and there are many, even now, who still maintain this approach could have worked if the execution had been better.

More-informed individuals subsequently told me that repeated waves were inevitable from the outset. They knew that by sheer virtue of the speed and extent of the spread, this new infection would be impossible to tame. But at this time I thought Covid would die out and not come back. Perhaps I looked for more optimistic viewpoints, whether these were of the 'the worst is already over' variety or the 'if we just suppress for long enough, we can eliminate it completely' variety. Or maybe I just couldn't take on the reality emotionally and therefore I mentally rejected future waves out of hand. I do know that I clung to this belief like a life raft: if I could just hold on and keep treading water, the wreckage of my business could be rebuilt, and I could carry on as before. I was also falsely reassured by the fact that the CBILS, announced at the beginning of April, was designed to cover six months of costs. My conclusion was that the government expected it to be over by then.

By the end of April, I had applied for and received my CBILS loan. This process was surprisingly smooth. Having received my application and supporting documentation, a Barclays Bank worker called me on Easter Monday, a bank holiday, to finalise the approval. Rather than challenging me on affordability (impossible for me to defend), she made sure I had included all my fixed costs in the proposal. I borrowed more than I had originally set out to do, something for which I would be very grateful in the following months.

Twitter was, and still is, an often-hostile environment, but once I had time to breathe, I found it essential. News articles and scientific papers appeared here first, and when I had time I would try to gain clues about what would happen next and how to plan for it. I searched for anyone involved in policy, followed scientists, journalists and academics, and asked questions to both improve my understanding and campaign for my business. As time went on I realised people were not concerned about the harms of lockdown in the same way I was, so I started to try to communicate my specialist knowledge into the mix. I found a community of professionals and private individuals who shared my concerns but from different specialist and personal perspectives. This group was invaluable to me: not only did

I learn from them, but they helped me feel less alone. Knowing that other people felt the same made me realise I wasn't delusional and helped me to feel rather less of a failure. My business was a disaster, online schooling for the children was far from ideal, and I felt like I was drowning in responsibility. But Twitter is a brutal, unforgiving place. I wish I'd had the self-control to step back from it more: communicating concerns would lead to torrents of abuse until I learned to block the worst offenders or walk away when feeling angry and upset.

It was clear, of course, that physically isolating us from each other made it much more difficult to understand or have sympathy for other people's circumstances. The print and television news focused on the reproduction rate, the availability of PPE (personal protection equipment), PCR (polymerase chain reaction) tests and pressure on hospitals, not on the unintended collateral damage of lockdown. I wonder if we were misled by the availability of technology into believing we were rather more connected than we were.

When we gathered around the television for the daily bulletin, it felt like it should have been our Churchillian moment: huddling around the radio to hear a rousing wartime speech, united against a common enemy. But for me this sense of 'being in it together' failed to materialise. The messaging seemed to set us against each other by blaming those who didn't or couldn't comply with restrictions to limit the virus's continued spread, and without the camaraderie of in-person social contact, there was little to offset it.

Whilst the use of such strong messaging seemed intended to shock us quickly into compliance, I couldn't help but be horrified by it. And it wasn't long before neighbourhood curtains started twitching. Both traditional and social media showed people reporting each other to the police for going out more than once a day. For some, a virtue was made of not leaving home at all.

Healthy households held on to their delivery slots rather than picking their food themselves. They ordered from online retailers to alleviate the boredom, without reflecting that they'd passed their risk on to the warehouse workers and delivery drivers. These same retailers quickly moved to ban third-party marketplace businesses from using their infrastructure, and without this, with retail shops closed, many businesses could not trade at all.

I was surprised there wasn't more outrage about this. Instead, we had 'non-essential' aisles of supermarkets taped off. No solution was found to help keep UK-based, bricks-and mortar-businesses trading. There were reliefs and handouts to help with costs, of course: a year without business rates if your premises were small enough and a grant of £25,000 if your business was within a sector compelled to close. And after a few weeks came the furlough scheme to save the jobs of those employed by you (who would otherwise have been made redundant) together with coronavirus business loans. But those who conducted their business through a limited company had no income support at all. Those who worked for limited companies were in a much better position than the companies themselves.

Of course, I know others were going through worse. I didn't lose anyone. I wasn't working in an intensive care unit. People will feel that I was lucky by comparison, and I was. I clapped on the doorstep, not for one group of people but for everyone. I knew how much I was struggling. I didn't want to struggle; I didn't choose it. I wondered what others were going through. I knew I had slipped through the net. The support groups for limited companies showed me there were millions more in my position, and many of them didn't have the good fortune to fall back on their partner for financial support.

I also know others suffered less; one of my patients told me she'd had a 'lovely lockdown'. Some enjoyed having their family around and seeing more of their husbands. Many saved money. Some enjoyed the absence of a long commute and welcomed the opportunity to roam in the countryside. Some on furlough enjoyed a fabulous barbecue summer: a paid sabbatical. I am aware that for some this was far from the reality, but for me it felt like a bribe to ensure compliance. I didn't blame those people for their good fortune or my lack of it, and I hoped I would be magnanimous enough to feel compassionate about their loss when this changed again. But I really couldn't stand the barrage of perfect home schooling or 'what to do when you're bored' articles in the papers and on social media.

Many seemed to assume that small businesses had a great deal of help. This is how it worked for me in practice.

1. Government

In my opinion furlough saved jobs, not businesses (furlough refers to the Coronavirus Job Retention Scheme, with the UK government paying up to 80% of employees' salaries). My business didn't qualify for the reliefs offered to other sectors, so I didn't receive a grant or any business rates relief. Those with limited companies who took their pay in dividends had no support with their income. In March 2020 I was accruing debt at the rate of £5,000 per week without pay. The only shining light was my local MP, Nickie Aiken, who campaigned on my behalf. I feel sure she influenced the eventual release of discretionary grant money for local councils to consider businesses on a case-by-case basis. At the beginning of April 2020, the government announced that the CBILS loan would be extended to businesses that could otherwise secure regular commercial loans. This was much more attractive than a commercial loan: not only was it at a much lower interest rate (3.5% above the Bank of England's base rate, then at 1%) but it did not require a personal guarantee. There would be a six-month holiday before starting repayments, and no interest would be charged for the first year. The government would underwrite a large proportion of the loan and pay for the first year of interest, allowing banks to offer more favourable terms.

2. Professional Body

The CSP (Chartered Society of Physiotherapy) had its hands full coping with the stress on NHS acute services. Anyone struggling in the private sector was advised to try to get a job in the NHS. Many of us joined the NHS bank but were never used. The CSP was silent about our rapid descent into debt, even when NHS employees received a 4.6% pay rise and an additional 6%+ in employer's pension contributions in June 2020. The CSP eventually helped with recommendations on reopening but then threw all its weight into campaigning for an enhancement to the NHS 1% pay rise.

3. Medical Insurance Companies

With a couple of exceptions, they ruthlessly exploited the opportunity to drive traffic towards their services. Many insurers are both referrers and providers, and policyholders wanting a different service or choice of practitioners pay more for the privilege. But this choice was denied to many. The insurance companies played hardball, and you could only fight this by using every single tool available, including patients. And even when an agreement was reached, one company took three further weeks to provide billing codes, putting an additional cash-flow crisis on top of the huge drop in income.

4. Business Interruption Insurance

The insurance company refused to pay out, even though I had an unspecified infectious disease clause. The government didn't tell us to shut, our professional body did, and my policy clearly stated the cover would only apply if we had been told to close by the chief medical officer. The only way my cover would kick in would be if I had a confirmed case of Covid at the practice. I produced evidence of my illness, but since Covid hadn't caused my business to close at the time of my illness, they still refused to pay.

5. Landlord

The Barbican Estate couldn't have been nicer. Although I still paid my March 2020 bill, they gave me the next quarter free and directed me towards other grants that might be available.

6. Local Council

This didn't start well. The local council took my April 2020 rates bill out early, which threw me into an overdraft. They agreed to staged business rates payments but offered no reduction. But they came up trumps, eventually, by awarding me grants totalling the amount I would have had at the outset had I been in retail, hospitality or leisure.

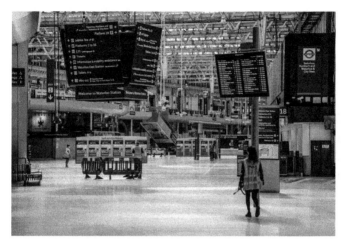

London stations at rush hour, Lockdown 1.

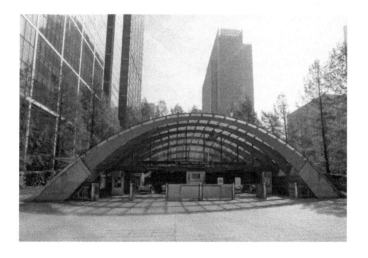

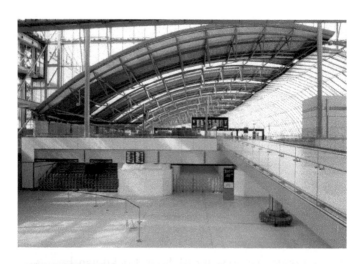
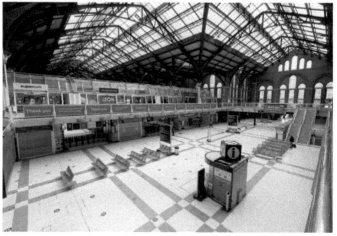

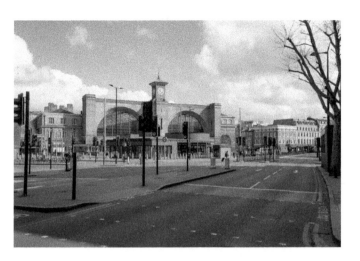

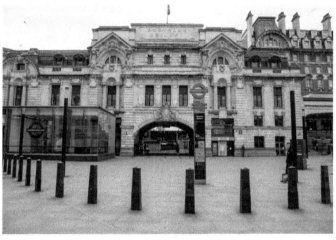

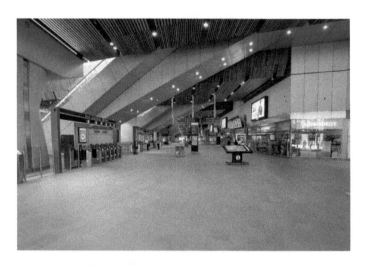

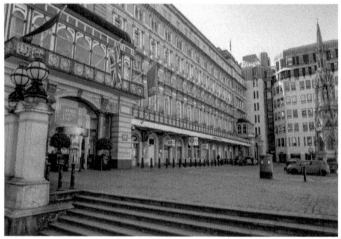

5 Reasons To Be Fearful: Part One

Outside my business concerns, I worried about the health effects of lockdown because I know that the maintenance of good health is effortful, not effortless. Even when we don't recognise it as such. Many behaviours can become habitual and unnoticed – normalised. So much so that we take their beneficial effects for granted. For my cohort of office workers, I worried specifically about working from home.

Commuting has numerous health benefits. Take the physical act of leaving your home: many people don't think of this as anything other than an irritation. They put in their headphones, walk to the station and walk to their office at the other end. They say hello to the receptionist and their colleagues, smile at a friend in the corridor and ask people how they are. All these individual activities, and more, confer mental and physical health benefits.

The transition between home and work allows you to switch on mentally for the tasks ahead. On the way back home, you can reflect on the events of the day and start to wind down. By commuting, not only do you physically leave work, but by association, you mentally leave work too. This gives an opportunity to unwind from the stresses of the day, relax in the evening and sleep well at night.

When commuting you change position repeatedly. Sometimes even those who drive to work will walk around more at work than they would do at home. A mini, unrecognised, cardiovascular workout as you breathe more deeply during the transition. Your muscles contract and move your body, maintaining joint and muscle health.

Without the ability to wind down and relax, I was concerned that those whose stress was already a risk factor for illness would see their health deteriorate. Emotional stress stimulates the sympathetic nervous system function of fright, flight and fight, increasing heart rate and blood pressure and diverting blood to the peripheral muscles, ready to run away from danger. In contrast the parasympathetic nervous system of relax, repair and renew allows your body to recover. Not only to repair the damage but also to prepare for the next burst of sympathetic activity. It's one of the reasons we need to sleep: turning off the mental override allows our systems to repair.

Stress-related illnesses occur when this balance is lost: the sympathetic system is fired up by an increase in mental activity, overriding repair mechanisms and disturbing sleep. There is a strong relationship between stress and illness for this reason: stress causes more inflammation and suppresses the function of the immune system, which is a parasympathetic process. This is why fear and anxiety are so damaging to health.

It is my professional experience that most people have a weak link: the first thing to go wrong when this balance is disturbed. For some it is migraine, for some neck pain, and for some irritable bowel syndrome. I often think of this as a flag that the balance has been lost, rather than blaming the specific source of symptoms in isolation. Illness and injury can be opportunistic, only causing problems when health and dominant pathways are disarmed by environmental stressors. These protective layers of healthy experience are stripped away by a more inflammatory sympathetic overload, and the pathways of previous conditions are uncovered, causing symptoms once again.

For my cohort of white-collar office workers, I was worried that those with existing or chronic conditions would see these worsen with a lack of commuting. I suspected they were unlikely to make up the difference with other exercise or techniques to switch on and off for the working day. Whilst they might make the effort to go running or take an online class, I feared this was likely, at best, to replace the exercise they weren't getting from their gym or pool. And, of course, the mental on–off switch would be absent.

I also feared that those who didn't have problems, but who had multiple risk factors, might find that the removal of their inadvertent coping mechanisms would throw them into illness states that would be difficult to recover from. If you have multiple risk factors, once the balance is tipped into illness, there may be no absolute cure, and these conditions can easily become permanent. Once suffered, even a minor, spontaneously resolving condition cannot be unsuffered. You cannot unpull the trigger or unshoot the gun. You can't 'not have had' it. This is why prevention is always better than cure. And why I feared that restriction-related harms would not be easy to unwind.

Established lifestyle-related illnesses do not subside by simply undoing the triggers that caused them. Once there, the brain models new pathways to create a new default mechanism, like an errant pacemaker, firing up neurones and perpetuating illness. Recovery can sometimes occur if new pathways of experience start to crowd out the pathways of illness. Layers and layers are built around this harm, making it comparatively smaller and less dominant over time. You create and reinforce a new normal, and the brain remodels around that instead. However, you do not recover if illness pathways continue to be elicited, or if there hasn't been sufficient time to allow new, healthier pathways to dominate. Nor do you recover if your body isn't allowed the time to heal: overriding your symptoms by force of will results in, at best, a longer recovery and, at worst, chronic illness.

Although I was concerned for my office workers, outside work I was much more worried for those most vulnerable to restrictions: the very young and the very old. Early and later life provide unique vulnerabilities. In the young, who have rapidly developing bodies and minds, there are periods of hyper development, so-called 'critical periods', during which time there is a huge proliferation of white matter in the brain. These periods allow the development of fundamental, basic pathways. Our rules for living. For example, from birth to three years of age many of the pathways of emotional attachment and language development are laid down. Once these proliferative phases have passed, it is extraordinarily difficult to override and recalibrate; they will always be present as the first response, even if extraordinary measures have managed to eclipse them.

The challenge in later life is to slow down the descent into frailty. Death occurs in most when function decays to such an extent that it is incompatible with life. Minor illnesses will result in, at best, a return to the same point on the descent, but they often cause an acceleration of frailty. If an old person is close to the line, minor illness may result in them crossing it; though if they are this vulnerable, the cause of death will not be primarily the acute illness, but rather what caused them to be frail in the first place.

The lack of understanding around the multifactorial composition of good health and ill health has been a barrier to objective critical thinking around the wisdom of imposing restrictions. The key to living and quality of life is to be as healthy as possible. Locking up our frail citizens (by telling them to shield) and closing schools would inevitably cause a great deal of damage. Those vulnerable to Covid might also be harmed by being told to shield: lack of access to exercise, lack of good food and lack of social contact would make them less well and less able to fight off

Covid or any other illness. This is why I, as a physiotherapist, had reasons to be fearful.

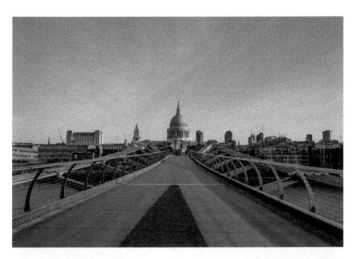

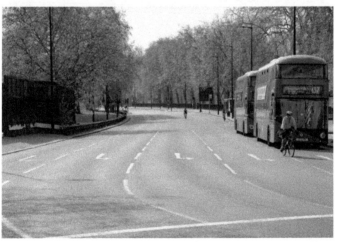

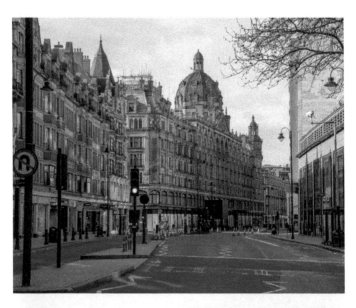

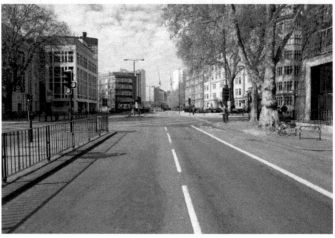

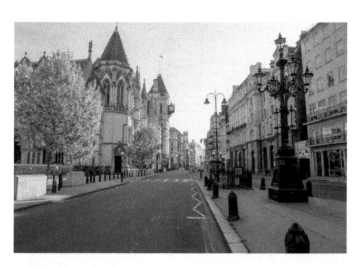

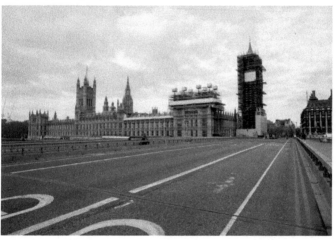

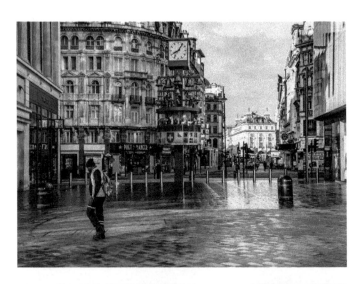

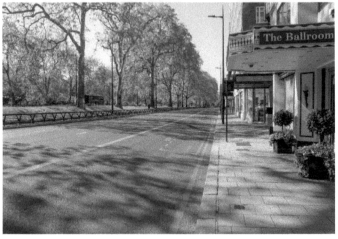

6 London in Lockdown

I do not aspire to country living. To begin with, it seems to require an extraordinary amount of driving, and I hate driving. And as much as I'd love a garden and however much I enjoy long walks in beautiful places, the boredom of having so little to do when the rain falls is a deal breaker for me. What I love is the buzz of a city. The way it constantly reinvents itself. New restaurants to try, theatre shows to watch, art exhibitions to see and people to meet. My happiness and well-being thrive on new experiences; my relaxation is dependent on distraction, not introversion.

My life is punctuated by the discovery of the new and the celebration of the old. This superficially ever-changing metropolis maintains its constant spirit – a living, breathing collection of history and memories – in the fabric of its buildings and even in the strata of rock beneath its buildings. Boudicca's layer of reddish-brown ash and broken Roman pottery (the residues of the torching of London in AD61) still lie beneath us. The excavations for new buildings are regularly paused at the discovery of Roman settlements beneath. I loved reading Peter Ackroyd's *London, A Biography*, with his description of rivers as the arteries and veins of this city's beating heart.

London has been attacked repeatedly by war, fire and famine, and yet it has always recovered, though some scars have healed more beautifully than others. Unfortunately, the choices made by London's custodians have sometimes appeared to be shaped by ego, rather than the desire to create spaces people will want to live or work in. To me, some of the newer city buildings look like competitive phalluses: I remain unsure if this is a fitting analogy of a dog-eat-dog corporate mindset, or rather a triumph of the 'can we' over the 'should we' mentality of architectural vanity. Similarly, the sweeping glass and steel of South Bank apartment blocks from the praying mantis of St George's Wharf eastwards seem competitive, but only in their vulgarity. The 'sky-high' pool of exclusivity located in the Embassy Gardens Estate offers a suitable viewing platform to look down on those unblessed by extreme wealth and the narcissism that seems too often to accompany it. Thankfully, the regeneration of other areas has been more successful, and many discoveries inspire delight over distaste.

Since moving to London in 1987, I have lived mostly in different areas of south London. But in 2007, just before our first child was born, my husband and I moved to Pimlico. Unfamiliar to many, Pimlico lies between the Thames and Buckingham Palace Road with Chelsea to the west, Westminster to the east and Belgravia to the north. In the middle lie Thomas Cubitt's white, stucco-fronted Victorian houses, arranged into the Pimlico Grid and now protected as a conservation area. On the periphery you find Peabody housing estates and Churchill Gardens, the latter being a large, sprawling council estate just north of the river, built after the Second World War. Lupus Street, running between the estate and the Pimlico Grid, is an eclectic mix of hardware stores, chemists and different types of specialised food shops.

Workwise I was still in the thick of it. Thankfully, the furlough scheme had been announced, as had the CBILS business loan scheme. My company wasn't at imminent risk of collapse, instead I had an enormous amount of long-term debt. There was still a lot to do to plan the reopening (when permitted) and make sure our online service was working smoothly.

I was uncomfortable with online consultations and keen to return to seeing patients in person. I just wasn't sure if I was able to diagnose accurately online. Even though I learn the most about someone's condition from taking their history, I still use touch to check my hypotheses, to treat and to teach. Sending someone out of my treatment room with less pain and more confidence in performing physical tasks is a big part of the job for me. I also gain a lot from observing how comfortably people move and what positions they assume when talking. This non-verbal communication is a key part of my examination, and without it, I felt uneasy.

I would try to ensure no harm could come from mistakes made in online consultations by sending emails with caveats and videos of exercises. This would usually take more time than the appointment itself, but we were hardly overloaded with patients, and it was my professional responsibility to do the best I could with an untested medium. It felt like we had embarked on a massive trial without a control group, and we didn't know how long it would run for. We were making the best of it, but I was convinced we were fooling ourselves that this method of consultation was anywhere near as effective as it was in person.

Most of the wealthy residents of central London had decamped to their country of origin or their second home, leaving parts of it eerily quiet. Around Victoria, the homeless were the only constant presence on the streets, and every day they gathered and sat in the sunshine on the steps outside the Apollo Victoria Theatre. Pimlico felt post-apocalyptic. I was used to weaving my way through crowded streets, looking four or five people ahead to spot the dawdling tourists and find gaps to squeeze through. I knew all the cut-throughs and when the lights changed at every busy junction. In April 2020 it was a ghost town.

There was no traffic, not even parked cars in the usually crowded residents' bays. There were very few people living this centrally, and the main roads were wide and silent. The wind whistled, unbuffered by the resistance of moving parts, and the streets bounced the reflected sound as efficiently as a tiled bathroom. Instead of plotting my path through the chaos, I looked up. I saw signs on the sides of buildings directing me to ancient bathhouses. Previously unnoticed, pretty casement windows or blue plaques speaking the names of famous past residents. Window boxes, mostly empty like the houses they adorned, but occasionally bursting with the colour of tulips or late daffodils.

I was told that other areas were very different. In some suburban areas of London, most of the shops were essential, so they stayed open. And people living there were not, in general, those who could work from home. Reducing community transmission through locking down seemed unlikely to have any effect here: these people all had to work in person. All this activity was essential; these residents were the supermarket workers, the care workers, the cleaners, the porters and the security guards. These were people who died in disproportionately high numbers during the first wave. And their communities were a densely packed hive of essential contacts.

Wealthy areas outside the centre were busy too. Instead of commuting, city workers stayed at home. Pavements and parks were full of those taking their one daily session of permitted exercise; some parks were even temporarily closed due to overcrowding.

Back in Westminster, my thirteen-year-old and I walked past the people queueing around the block for Sainsbury's and headed to a supermarket on Cardinal Place, which was surrounded by shuttered offices and where the queues were non-existent. (We had quickly discovered the best-stocked shops were in areas where people worked rather than where they lived.) Approaching the Apollo Victoria Theatre steps, we saw two men less than ten feet away from us enter a phone box and inject themselves in the forearm. Without even bothering to shut the door. Quite a change from the usual immaculate social media influencers posing for photos beside these same iconic landmarks.

5 April 2020 was a memorable day with late spring sunshine and a smattering of fluffy white clouds. We decided to walk up to Trafalgar Square, Leicester Square and Piccadilly Circus via St James's Park, remembering to walk in single file and at least two metres away from anyone we came across (and having to remind the children repeatedly to do this too).

At the tourist landmarks there were many discarded bikes, with their riders taking photos of the now-empty bits of central London.

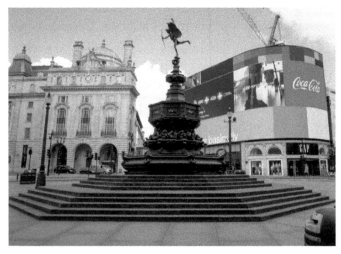

Piccadilly Circus 5th April 2020

I ventured into Tesco on Jermyn Street, having seen someone leave with a rare bag of bread flour. I was delighted to find not only bread flour but also yeast. When I left the shop, my husband was talking to a couple of police officers who had blocked his path with their van. He was being told off. According to one police officer, we were not taking exercise because he had a large SLR camera with him. According to the police officer we were sightseeing, especially as we weren't wearing Lycra.

The police officers asked us where we had come from. The answer was Victoria, which was a twenty-minute walk away. 'You have to understand, Madam, that people are coming in from Zone Six.' (Zone Six refers to the outer range of the public transport fare zone of London, approximately twelve to sixteen miles from Piccadilly Circus.)

'Hmm, well, we live in Victoria. We haven't sat on the grass or a park bench. We haven't touched anything, in fact, and I have not allowed my children to bring out a ball or a kite. We are trying to make it interesting for them.'

'Well, Madam, we have seen you walking around taking photos for the last ten minutes.'

'OK, we will go home then.'

'Oh, you don't have to go straight home.'

'I don't understand; I thought you were telling us we were doing something wrong?'

I'm still not sure whether they felt they couldn't backtrack or whether they still thought we were in the wrong. I told them again that, as a family, we were trying to make ethical, responsible choices and avoid our closest park, Battersea Park, because it was so busy. And as a physiotherapist, I felt entitled to decide what the definition of exercise was. They let us be.

On our way back through St James's, the Metropolitan Police were out in full force. People were sitting on the grass, and everyone was very diligent about maintaining their space. It wasn't difficult: there must have been fewer than one hundred people in the whole park. Two police officers approached a couple who were batting a shuttlecock between them and their two-year-old. They told the family to move along. The police swept through the park, an advancing line of them, crushing this brief pleasure of such a beautiful day, like a wave over a sandcastle.

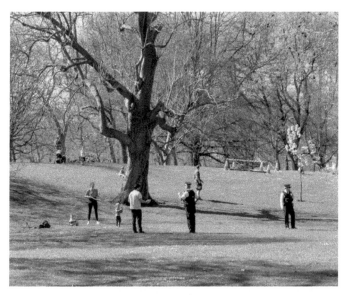

St James's Park 5th April 2020

We were challenged repeatedly by police officers in that first lockdown. I had the feeling that some who did so enjoyed the sense of power. Not a good time to be living in the city centre with children and no garden.

Other trips were more successful. On one occasion we found one of our favourite restaurants, The Oystermen in Covent Garden, selling food supplies from the window. Andrea, the manager, greeted us like long-lost family, and we staggered home with an eclectic mix of fresh produce, ingredients and antipasti. A similarly successful trip was a long walk up to Abbey Road Studios, getting 'that' zebra crossing photo with nobody else in the frame and finding a

Lebanese restaurant, Noura, open for takeaway food on the way back. We feasted like kings that day.

These surprise discoveries, unexpected but simple pleasures, gave us reason and justification within the law to leave the house and be able to entice the children out too. What had first happened by chance soon happened by design. We toured London on foot, avoiding the police presence in parks, to find deserted tourist areas and the occasional store selling delicious takeaway food.

What was notable in that first lockdown was the friendliness of those we met. Londoners have a reputation for being rude and unwelcoming, but everyone was charming. My husband took to sitting outside our front door 'on the stoop' watching the world go by and briefly chatting with those returning from their permitted walk or food shop. The weather was glorious throughout that first lockdown. Through the NHS clap we learned to recognise neighbours we hadn't known previously, as we can see at least ten doorsteps from our own.

The advice on masks had changed dramatically. To begin with, most counselled against them, advising they might do more harm than good by providing a false sense of security. But when the main mode of transmission was thought to be via droplets, people started to wear them. I mean, it made sense, didn't it? The droplets would be caught in the cloth masks, whilst air was allowed to pass through.

All medical-grade masks had been diverted into the NHS, so my younger daughter and I found some modelling wire and made a mould of our faces. I revised the musculature of the cheeks, knowing that a good fit would be key to preventing the moisture from leaking out around the edges of our masks. (We still thought at that stage that the virus could live for a while on any surface it touched.) We were quite pleased with the result and wore our masks religiously on our daily outside walks.

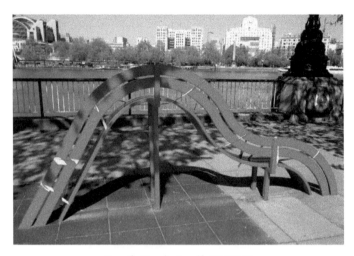

South Bank April 19 2020

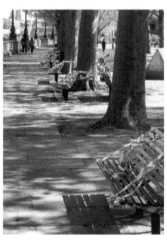
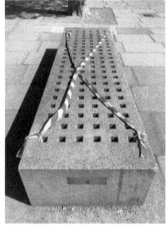

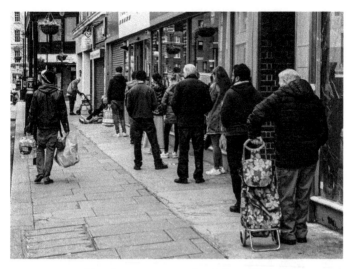

Food store queues Lockdown 1.

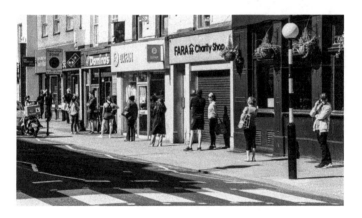

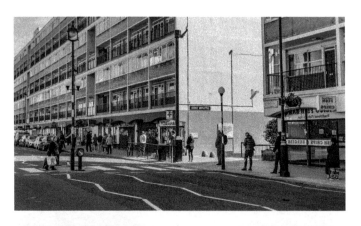

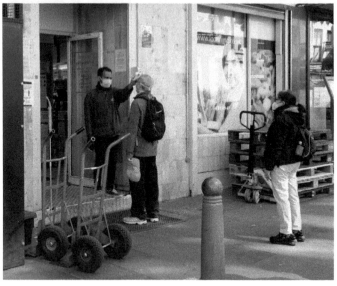

7 My Crash (and Burn) Course in Post-Viral Illness

By May restaurants had started opening for deliveries, many with long queues of Deliveroo cyclists waiting outside. We collected ours in person from those restaurants that allowed it. On one occasion this was a gorgeous dim sum lunch from Royal China on Baker Street, which we gobbled down whilst sitting in the sunshine at the northern end of Hyde Park. Much to the envy of passers-by.

We didn't have a dog, but we started taking our drinks for a walk instead. We couldn't get hold of any tonic water or lemons, so we had gin, a wedge of orange and soda water in thermos flasks designed for coffee. (There was a widespread shortage of soft drinks.) We walked around our neighbourhood in the lengthening evenings, hoping to see friends, to see anything interesting, just to have something to experience other than the inside of our house. One couple we knew would sit by their open front window every Friday and Saturday night and welcome a series of visitors. Their children sat just inside their front door, with ours standing on the street, discussing just how weird their lives had become.

One time we stayed longer than usual until we became ravenously hungry. As luck would have it, one of the pubs on Warwick Way was selling fish and chips through the window, with ale sold in two-litre plastic milk jugs to wash it down. For the first time since lockdown had been announced, there was a bit of a buzz. With the lighter evenings, people started taking their constitutionals later, almost like the Italian *passagiata*, though, of course, we were banned from sitting down, and the public loos were still closed.

My younger daughter had her tenth birthday. In an attempt to celebrate it, we made and hand-delivered cupcakes to her friends, meeting over Zoom to chat and sing happy birthday. Sadly, it was more of a reminder of what was missing than it was a celebration: in hindsight we should have just written it off. But at least she saw her friends in person, at a distance, when we delivered the cakes.

I joined the Serpentine Swimming Club in Hyde Park, which allowed me to swim in a cordoned-off area of the lake, the Serpentine Lido. Sitting in the sunshine on the bank and watching the birds swim up and down was a very refreshing change, even if I did almost swim into a swan on more than one occasion. But having suffered a nasty bite on my throat from something lurking in the water, and with an awareness that I still hadn't fully recovered from Covid, I stopped after five or six visits. Avoiding the swans was quite entertaining in one sense though, and at least I had done something different. It was a thirty-minute walk from home; walking up Sloane Street to Knightsbridge and through Hyde Park was another unique, echoed 'empty-London' experience.

I still didn't feel well. The cough had gone, finally, but I just couldn't get going. My back was sore, and I had constant sciatic pain through working long hours from my bed. I needed to move, and walking wasn't enough. But a two-mile run or a visit to the lido would have me in bed the next day, so exhausted I could barely lift my head. I realised that this wasn't normal fatigue, it was post-viral. And for post-viral fatigue the medicine is rest, not exercise.

To help my back and sciatic pain, I devised a set of exercises and started changing my working position more regularly: all standard advice I would give my patients. It didn't solve the problem, but it made it tolerable. I was still working very hard, but it was more manageable now. And once we were able to start treating in person at the end of May, and I had set up my Covid-safe measures, there was less administration for me to do.

I started asking questions on social media about ME (myalgic encephalomyelitis), recovery from viral illnesses and post-intensive care syndrome. I read an enormous number of medical papers to try to figure out how to signpost any patients who came with musculoskeletal pain, but who may have had Covid. I knew I couldn't rehabilitate them normally, since trying this myself had clearly given me PEM (post-exercise malaise), which is a marker of ME – a persistent post-viral illness characterised by extreme fatigue.

I learned about energy envelopes, pacing, PoTS (postural tachycardia syndrome) and anaerobic thresholds. I watched webinars, and I started to figure out how to avoid making people worse. I learned that PEM could be caused not only by physical exercise but also by mental exercise. I will always be grateful to those who were patient with me at that time. PhysiosForME webinars were clear, comprehensive and practically applicable. I developed some guidelines on how to identify patients who needed to be referred. I also developed guidelines on how to try to prevent these syndromes by getting enough rest in the early stages, becoming aware that people often felt better before feeling worse again. I advocated for my patients with their employers and started advising the companies I worked with. And anything I gave patients, even without prior symptoms of fatigue, would be within the amount of exercise they would do in one day, not on top of it.

With the realisation that cognitive exercise could contribute to fatigue and knowing the effect of stress on inflammation and pain, I started to advise patients not only to leave their residences for their allotted exercise (within their energy envelope if they had had Covid) but also to bookmark their day. Without commuting, I felt there was a need for something to allow patients to mentally gear up for work and then recover from it. Interestingly, the feedback I've had since has been that this simple strategy did more to relieve pain than any specific exercise, change of chair or other pieces of equipment I recommended.

But once the technology had been set up for home working, Zoom meetings and other work started to infiltrate what had previously been commute time. There became no division or compartmentalisation of work and home. Because of lockdown there was an assumption that people were always available, and workers, anxious about their job security, felt compelled to oblige. It's no wonder that working from home quickly became, for some, like living at the office.

Setting work boundaries could simply consist of going to the corner shop for a pint of milk, changing clothes or listening to music. It didn't need to be exercise. And whilst they were working, patients were advised to change positions, taking thinking time to lie down with arms outstretched or to make a cup of tea. I'd highlight research showing that this would make them more productive, not less. I'd advise patients to make video calls only on audio where possible, allowing them to pace around the room or lie down – anything to change position without adding to their physical or mental burden.

I started to ask on Twitter if some patients might benefit from a graded rehabilitation strategy. I hadn't seen anyone clearly reporting PEM at this stage, but I saw plenty who had had Covid and developed musculoskeletal complaints. This was not a popular question, though I felt justified in asking it. My caseload was more likely to involve muscle and joint pain caused by a change in activity, rather than persistent viral symptoms: the most common complaints were spinal pain from increased sitting or knee pain in people who had taken up running. My intention was to ensure I didn't inadvertently cause other problems. In my role, but not in acute care, respiratory or neuro, I saw many patients who had had Covid but who didn't have PEM.

My clinical caseload consists of patients who work beyond their physical capabilities: high-achieving, driven individuals who are highly intelligent, uncomplaining and hardworking. The type of people who always meet their deadlines and who work when they are sick. These were the patients who had RSI (repetitive strain injury) or other work-related musculoskeletal pain, vulnerable because of their work ethic, their perfectionism and their drive to succeed. I had mentally earmarked this group (with more low-grade inflammation from the constant mental overriding of their body's needs) as being the most vulnerable to prolonged post-viral symptoms after Covid. I couldn't understand the response that insisted all was biomedical, and that work stress and personal circumstances couldn't be a contributing factor, since this went against everything I knew about dealing with patients who had persistent musculoskeletal pain.

In healthcare there is an ongoing debate between the biopsychosocial model and one of mind–body dualism. The former principle asserts that illness does not work in a vacuum: risk factors, severity and outcomes will depend on who is afflicted, not just on the nature of the diagnosis. Mind–body dualism suggests the condition is entirely biomedical, so the solution depends on the type and delivery of treatment and not on the response or characteristics of the patient or their environment.

This is the trap I had inadvertently fallen into. Post-viral syndromes are still poorly understood. Many patients have been disbelieved and have been told there was no biological cause for their complaint, and that there was solely a psychological cause leading to physical deconditioning, the implication being that they lacked the motivation to recover. Many had been put on rehabilitation programmes that made their condition dramatically worse.

But there was never any suggestion from me that post-viral conditions did not have a biological component, were a choice or were secondary to a lack of will or emotional strength – quite the opposite. My patients developed problems because of their emotional determination, not in spite of it. They had already tried to override their physical capabilities many times. That is why, when they did develop a problem, they put up with it for months before presenting. And my biggest challenge was always to persuade them to reduce their work time by prioritising the urgent and putting off what was not, whilst dealing with any mechanical cause for their symptoms and improving their resilience to further injury.

My own Long Covid, if that's what it was, settled after seven months. At that point I could gradually increase my exercise without crashing. A seemingly spontaneous, rapid recovery. All because, I believe, after my period of concentrated work to save the business, I'd given my body time to heal and time to clear the virus. I had dodged a bullet. I was very grateful for the advice I had received; it was clear to me that this extended period of relative physical rest had allowed my body to recover. I had prevented my body from turning on itself in the form of an autoimmune-driven illness. I was lucky that the mental stress and hard work hadn't caused me to develop a much longer, chronic, post-viral fatigue syndrome.

My concern grew that the core message of adequate recuperation (and enough sick leave) to prevent this secondary condition from developing would be lost. I was also concerned that much of the conversation seemed intent on proving Long Covid existed in large-enough numbers to justify a suppression strategy. It also seemed likely that the call for research would lead to the expectation that there was a single cause, a diagnostic marker that would result in a magic-wand, curative treatment. Sadly, I've worked in healthcare long enough to think that extremely unlikely.

My other concern was that graded exercise tolerance strategies would not be advised for those who would benefit from them. Every return to or increase in health and fitness involves a graded tolerance approach. If you want to run a marathon, you gradually increase your mileage. If you want to lift heavy weights, you start low and build up steadily. When people are ill, they should rest and slowly return to their work and exercise when they have cleared whatever illness sickened them. Occupational health departments devise a gradual return to work when employees have been off for some time. And so on.

Graded exercise tolerance is the right course of action, whether used formally or informally, for the majority of people in the majority of circumstances. That it doesn't suit those with PEM, or those who are yet to recover from acute illness, does not mean that it should be demonised as a strategy to return to full fitness for everyone else.

With the latent effects of lockdown making us progressively less healthy and fit, I worried that the addition of Covid would lead to an increasing rate of Long Covid diagnoses, when the cause of patients' symptoms primarily lay with the deterioration of their health beforehand. Restrictions had, for many people, started to reduce their resilience to illness, any illness, and worsen outcomes. I hoped that those with severe post-viral illnesses would get the advice and treatment they needed. But I also hoped that those needing an opposite approach would get what they needed too.

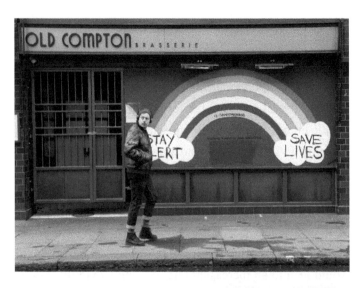

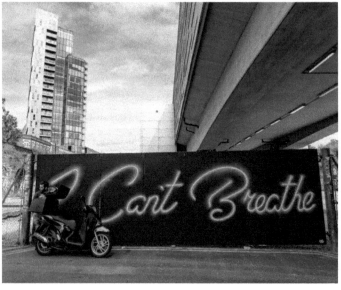

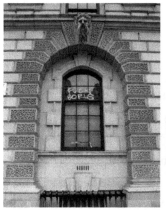 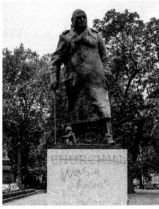

The day after the Black Lives Matter march of May 31 2020. This protest followed the killing of George Floyd by a US police officer.

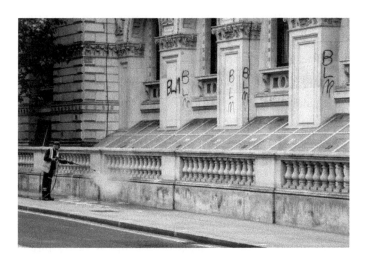

8 The Kids Are (Not) All Right

When schools first closed I assumed they'd reopen shortly after the Easter holiday. (They had been scheduled to return after the Easter break on 22 April.) But for most children, schools were closed for six months and were significantly limited for more than a year after that. At the start, home schooling had been an enjoyable novelty for some. Children were thrilled to be allowed more screen time. Our family was lucky enough to have the required technology from the outset, and both my children's schools made huge efforts to continue delivering the curriculum. I was a little concerned about removing all parental controls to run Teams, allowing them to source information from the internet, but we didn't have any choice; it seemed a minor gripe considering the circumstances.

But after two or three weeks of home schooling, learning loss was not the main concern. I spoke to parent after parent who reported that their children had started to change, becoming more insular and emotionally fractured. They missed their friends, their sport, their music and all their independence. Teachers insisted on cameras being turned on during live lessons. But this led to bullying: screenshots of briefly awkward expressions were circulated on WhatsApp groups, and there were taunting side chats on Teams. To see everyone's faces simultaneously without the opportunity of a side glance at a friend, whilst knowing you could be called upon at a moment's notice, was very difficult for many. And if you were caught out with a question, your discomfort would be seen by all – not so nurturing an environment for teenage girls.

Some children fared better than others. But for those I spoke to, particularly those in households without a spare adult to supervise, it was very difficult. For many, learning stopped being fun. Teachers may have been delivering excellent content, but it often wasn't received as these children increasingly switched off.

I had frequent conversations with other parents. Some more-introverted children, old enough not to need supervision, seemed to like online schooling. But these children became more and more withdrawn, almost agoraphobic. Far from leaving the house, they didn't want to leave their rooms, even to eat.

Other conversations revealed stories of older children, particularly girls, who really struggled and missed hanging out with their friends. In general, the boys seemed to cope better emotionally; they would game online in the same way they would game in person, looking at a screen rather than at each other. But they didn't want to go outside either. If they weren't allowed to take a football or meet a friend, where was the incentive? The playgrounds were forbidden and taped off too. The outside world was not very appealing to a miserable, lonely child.

Children simply started fading away. Turned their faces to the wall. Closed themselves off entirely. They didn't contact their friends much, even online, for what had they to discuss? Their inner lights turned off.

We already knew that technology, unless controlled by parents, could be devastating for the health and well-being of children. We started to get warning emails from school about predator networks attempting to groom our children.

I deleted my Facebook account after I was bombarded with all the evidence that I was failing as a parent: perfect home schooling and 'fun' craft homework, for example. I'm sure I wasn't alone in feeling irritated with this perfectly curated online life. Perhaps people were showing the world what they wanted to and were struggling too, but in my dark place it felt like mocking criticism.

Many newspaper columns dismissed any concern about the closure of schools, with commentators suggesting that this experience would give our children resilience. Whilst this may have been true for a small number of children living in otherwise privileged households, for other children this 'character building' was intolerable: we now know of the increase in anxiety, depression, anorexia and self-harm manifesting in this period. We also know that for some children home was not a safe place, but school, with its safeguarding processes, was. Politicians, scientists and journalists expressed concerns about learning loss, campaigning for laptops and free broadband, rather than the reopening of in-person schooling. Many suggested we should extend lockdown, including school closures, giving the reason that if we locked down for long enough, we wouldn't have to do it again.

Reading opinion after opinion, including those in the national press and medical journals, advocating for the continuation of school closures until we reached zero Covid, filled me with despair. From what I understood about childhood development and from what I had seen, I felt strongly that the opposite was true: it had become a moral and ethical obligation to find a way to reopen in-person schooling as soon as possible.

Musculoskeletal physiotherapists were allowed to start seeing patients face to face again at the end of May 2020 after risk assessment, the imposition of a one-way system, PPE, clinical waste collection and a Perspex screen for reception. The equipment required was in scarce supply and extremely expensive, though at least by then the PPE exchange had been set up, the NHS had sufficient supply, and I could get hold of some. I started going in two days a week, with the other three days earmarked for Test and Trace, which I'd been asked to do via the NHS bank. At my practice we trundled along seeing between twenty and thirty patients a week. Although we were allowed to work, the offices were still closed, so our only work came from the few local residents living in the commercial centre of town. The business was still losing money, but due to furlough this was £2,000 per week instead of the £5,000 it had been (although I was unable to furlough myself, as I still had to work).

With very little to do clinically, I offered our services to the local NHS GP at no charge for those who couldn't afford private practice but were not able to see anyone through the NHS. We could operate as a green zone – no Covid patients, with infection-control policy and risk assessment in place. I had useful skills, and it was very frustrating not to be able to use them. I asked similar questions of my professional body, but their response was to seek work through the NHS bank, rather than offering our private practices for NHS work.

The City and the commute were empty. If I went in early enough, my only companions in the train carriage were construction workers. If later, there would often be nobody at all. Despite that, it was rather lovely to get to work and see different faces even if they were, by then, masked.

When I returned to in-person work, I realised that for me there were limitations with online treatment. Of course, I could take a history in the same way, but anything requiring the confirmation of a physical examination was pretty hit-and-miss. This was particularly problematic when the patient hadn't been able to identify the cause or mechanism of injury, or when they assumed it was a recurrence of something they'd suffered previously. The very first person I treated on my return to work had improved with the general advice of the first session but not after the second. I realised by the time she sat down in front of me that my diagnosis had been wrong. It made me much more doubtful that the medium of online treatment would ever become the medium of choice, even with the benefit of ease of access.

Although private practices were not used for NHS work, the NHS bank did contact me to see if I'd be interested in applying to be a call handler for Test and Trace. The recruitment process was painful. Pages and pages of information, proof of identity, professional qualifications (usually checked online quickly and painlessly through our regulator's website), a half-hour online meeting with a recruiting nurse and an advanced DBS (disclosure and barring service) criminal records check. Then I had to download several different computer programs and run through security briefings, online clinical training and a series of induction processes related to safeguarding and internet security, amongst others.

I was to be a 'Tier Two': someone trained as a health care professional who could pick up calls the Tier Three team found difficult. The training was delayed by a week and took around sixteen hours to complete. I had been booked in for three eight-hour shifts per week. But I wasn't asked to make a single call in the first week. I hesitated to book more shifts, thinking this was a waste of public money, and then there were no shifts available to book. So, I stopped. I hadn't made a single call.

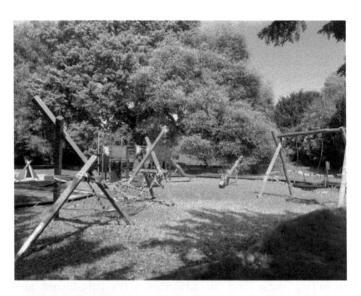

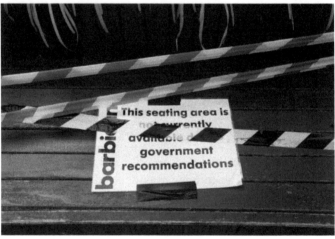

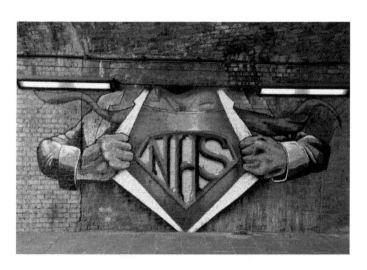

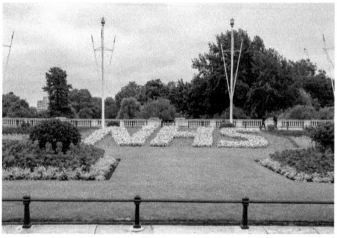

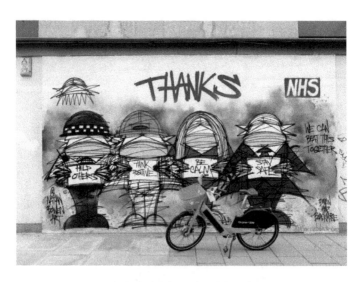
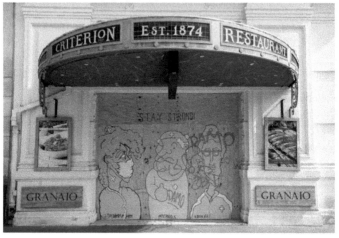

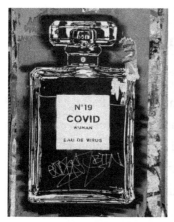
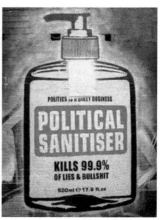
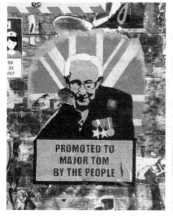
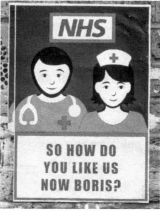

9 The Great Unlock of London

June had seen more restaurants opening for takeaways and in more imaginative ways than ever before. We had been back to Covent Garden and were delighted to find The Oystermen selling beer, oysters, and fish and chips from the window of the restaurant. Sitting on the pavement of Covent Garden piazza to eat it all, in full sunshine, was a moment of joyous indulgence.

I turned fifty on 1 July and managed a small get-together outside in Eccleston Yards – a secret, tucked-away courtyard haven in what was previously a power station. It felt awkward, slightly naughty, but oh so lovely. We had two groups of six people standing separately, and I ignored the guidance to move between the two. Fortunately, and coincidentally, there was a temporary gazebo for shelter when the rain came.

For the rest of July and August, London saw a progressive unwinding of restrictions.

On 4 July pubs and restaurants reopened for table service. We were delighted to return to our favourite local. That first pint of beer was the best pint I had ever tasted, and it was such a beautiful sunny day. We were welcomed like family by the landlord, who told us his business had lost a staggering £1,000,000, with his hopes of buying a home completely lost.

Covent Garden and the West End had been transformed. Westminster Council had agreed to allow tables in the street, and traffic was suspended. Tables spilled out from every restaurant. It felt very continental, and we hoped this was here to stay.

We started visiting art galleries too. Our first visit, to the Titian exhibition at The National Gallery, was quite extraordinary. There was nobody there. Well, a small, distanced queue outside, of course. But once inside we drank in the unique opportunity to sit in front of these great works with, at most, one or two other people in the room. We sought out our favourite artists on our extended private view: Rembrandt, Velasquez and more, without needing to be mindful of others waiting to view them and without the loud commentary of some uninvited amateur tour guide. We could allow all our senses to be engaged in the messages that lay within: Rembrandt's self-portraits seemed particularly poignant in the solitude of an empty room.

All the activities we loved about the city, but which had been forbidden to us, had started to return. And with no crowds. There were no tourists. We took full advantage.

Although inside swimming pools stayed shut, more lidos opened. We loved swimming in the chilly water at Parliament Hill Lido, which did allow children, and we particularly enjoyed the ice creams afterwards. (I didn't miss the Serpentine swans, or their excrement if I'm honest.)

People started returning to London, thirsty for company and hungry for variety.

Despite regular reminders and continued messaging, it felt as though we could start to look forwards and hope there would be an end soon. We felt emotionally battered, wanting to recover from what had been a truly dreadful episode in our lives.

We weren't ready to trust it, but there was a sense that the worst was over.

August was fabulous. Having known I'd had Covid and exposed my family to it, we had no hesitation in booking holidays. Of course, everything in the UK was very expensive and booked up a long time in advance but going abroad was ridiculously cheap. We managed a late booking to Rome, flying with British Airways for four nights in a four-star hotel next to the Trevi Fountain, for the cost of a night's stay in Cornwall. Rome was boiling hot – forty degrees centigrade – and empty. There were no queues at the Sistine Chapel, the Pantheon, the Villa Borghese, the Colosseum, or the Gelato de San Crispino, much to my children's delight.

In my favourite Roman place to revisit, the Villa Borghese, some of the greatest works are tucked away in the corner of a room. On previous visits I was always satisfied with gazing at Bernini's statue of *Apollo and Daphne*, wondering at the skill and vision required to depict her metamorphosis in such an unforgiving medium. Other works, such as those by Caravaggio, were always surrounded by hordes of people, and I lacked the patience to wait; I would only have wondered how long I could stay looking at them before it became rude not to let others have their turn. But this time there would be no crowd to alert me to the presence of these works, and I nearly missed them completely. What bliss, though, to sit for ten minutes on a studded leather bench with an uninterrupted view of *David and Goliath*.

We travelled to see friends we knew well in Liguria – an Italian resort where barely anyone spoke English but where everyone knew each other – having spent the summers together for decades. Our children were friends from school and could be independent in this safe place. They would go for pizza at 11 pm, coming back after midnight to find us still watching *padel* (a racket sport) outside the bar next to our hotel. One time my daughter was furiously typing away on Duolingo to figure out how to communicate with her new friends (and insult the boys), her face smeared with ice cream and decorated with a smattering of sand. The memory warms my heart.

The look of happiness on their faces by the end of this trip was such a relief. They laughed without hesitancy; previously furrowed brows were now smooth. I was so, so grateful to our dear friends, and when we came back it felt like our tank was full. We spent several evenings simply happy to be surrounded by the 'burble, burble' of Italian chatter and conviviality. Our friends were, as ever, extremely generous with their time, and they were perfect hosts.

London continued to open up. The Royal Court Theatre and Colbert Bistro shared space in the middle of Sloane Square, setting up a bar, tables and chairs, and even pétanque. It was surreal: drinking a martini in what had previously been disused space in the middle of a busy roundabout. Albeit in one of London's most expensive neighbourhoods.

London's metamorphosis into a continental city continued.

EOTHO (Eat Out to Help Out) was another break from the intensity of stress and anxiety we had experienced since March. Restaurants had Covid measures in place with social distancing and the majority of diners seated outside. To be around others and enjoy the experience of eating in company, albeit distanced, felt emotionally and physically fortifying. Despite the distancing and the masking to use the loo, we were around other people again and we could hear laughter and enjoyment all around us.

I don't think enough has been made of how this hiatus made what was to follow more bearable. At the very least it felt like a break, an opportunity to nurture the pathways of relaxation through human contact, but perhaps it was also a preventative against the establishment of stress-related illness.

Perhaps EOTHO was also a way to encourage people out of their solitude and back to work: if you were going out for social reasons, you couldn't really object to returning to the office. But there was a suspicion that the government wanted workers to return to city centres for the sole purpose of saving city businesses and commercial rents. And why should they return? Many preferred working from home; they had more freedom, and productivity remained surprisingly high.

Some of the larger tech companies suggested they would be happy with a permanent, full-time working-from-home model. Some articles appeared predicting the death of the City: this was a new dawn, a societal change that was being compared to the industrial revolution. I was very doubtful; I had already seen some of the issues with online working versus in-person working. But I hoped my business wouldn't be utterly destroyed before they found this out.

EOTHO did keep many struggling hospitality businesses going. These were the good guys who had employed their staff and furloughed them when told to close, but who couldn't afford to keep them on when the support started to wind down. There were still very few tourists, so restaurants were only half-full at the start. Fortunately, they became much busier very quickly as people gradually and tentatively booked in and continued doing so.

There was soon a staff shortage, and every pub and restaurant would tell you about it. Foreign nationals, who couldn't work in lockdown, had gone back home and couldn't afford the cost of testing to return. Chefs and waiting staff were being poached, lured by high salaries from the very businesses who had ruthlessly ditched them when lockdown was imposed. Demand quickly outstripped supply.

But the overwhelming response we had from hospitality was one of relief. This initiative coaxed people out of their homes and saved their businesses. They had worked extraordinarily hard, spending a great deal of money they didn't have to become Covid compliant. They obeyed the rules punctiliously, installing one-way systems, Perspex screens and Covid app QR codes for Test and Trace purposes. And those who visited their establishments were happy to be out again. It was all smiles, laughter and friendliness that August.

I hoped and prayed it was over. I had to keep going emotionally. I was already £100,000 down due to lockdown and thought another wave would mean the end of my business and the livelihoods I was trying so hard to protect.

The UK government had started to unwind furlough. From August employers would have to pay employer's contributions (approximately 20% of gross pay), and the amount of pay the government pledged to cover would reduce further each month, with the scheme ending at the end of October 2020. (This was subsequently extended.)

Rishi Sunak, the Chancellor of the Exchequer at the time, justified this decision by asserting that the country couldn't afford to prop up 'zombie businesses'. This upset me. We were still functioning at a fraction of normal, people were still advised to work from home, and I was still losing £2,000 per week because of costs. And at the end of September, I would be pushed off the cliff once again.

I thought Covid was over, and although case numbers were creeping up, test positivity rates stayed very low. But in reality, I had been taken in by the eye of the storm. The worst was yet to come.

As test positivity rates started to rise, it was clear there would be a second wave. I had my head in my hands hoping we wouldn't need to lock down again, that somehow infection rates would be contained, that people would start to return to the city, that children would stay at school (with reduced restrictions) and that we would be allowed to thrive, not just survive. Sadly, it was clear pretty quickly that this was wishful thinking.

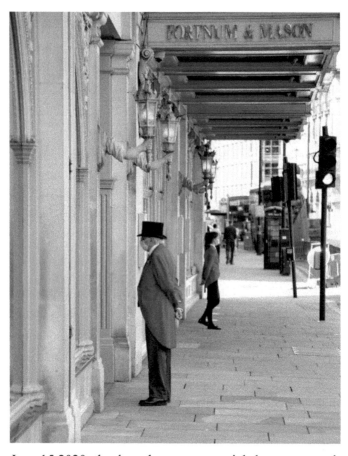

June 15 2020: the day when non essential shops reopened.

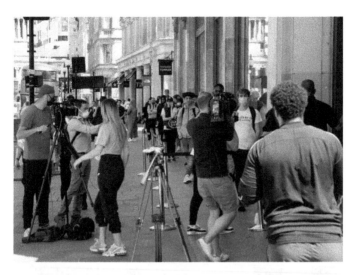
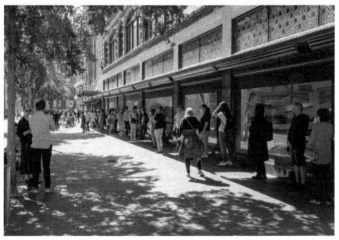

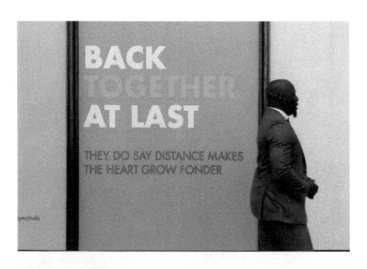
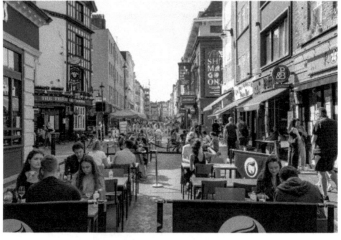

10 The Adults Aren't All Right Either

In September 2020 workers started to return to the City and my practice after six months of working from home. I had thought these people were the lucky ones: paid in full and able to work remotely. I was wrong, or at least, not entirely right.

I saw patients who hadn't been within two metres of another soul for six months. When I greeted them, they were tightly coiled springs, rigid with stress. They couldn't look me in the eye; they backed away and flinched when I touched them. I was utterly, utterly horrified.

Some told me they had been working more than fifteen hours a day from their beds. There had been no downward revision of productivity expectations: targets had to be met. With little else to do and scared of losing their jobs, they started work when they woke up, grabbing their laptops from beside their beds and only stopping to eat or go back to sleep. They were living at the office with no separation of home and work, and without being allowed any downtime at all. When coffee shops had opened for takeaways in May, some had visited them just to see another person, even if masked and at a distance.

This maintenance of productivity was celebrated as a new dawn of working, where the work–life balance would take precedence, using tech for everyone's benefit. Zoom and universal broadband access were sold as the modern-day version of the washing machine, liberating the laptop classes from the grind of their commute, and leaving time to enjoy life to the full.

But pre-pandemic advances in technology had already become a curse for many: whilst you could access your emails on the way home and at home, the ability to do so had meant for a long time that you were expected to work outside office hours. And on holiday. All these workplace mindfulness schemes seemed to me to miss the point. If you want your staff to be less stressed and take less time off sick, let them leave work and allow them some downtime. You can't have a work–life balance without life, and mental ill health was already an increasing problem.

I worried that the widespread adoption of video conferencing would make this worse. Whilst it should liberate, the time gained would inevitably be used for more work as companies sought to leverage this time to improve their performance in a highly competitive marketplace. And so it would prove to be.

What I wasn't prepared for was just how quickly I saw the results of this in my patients. For the first month or so, everyone was busy installing the infrastructure they needed, but as soon as that happened, this creep into social time began. Junior staff said they would find multiple Zoom meetings scheduled into their diaries, including during commute time, leaving them little time during the working day to do the job they were paid to do.

Many of the people I treated were foreign nationals cut off from their families or those who had moved to London to start work after university. Travelling home to families was banned, and they were living with virtual strangers in crowded flat shares. Or worse – alone – if their flatmates had managed to move home and work from there before the lockdown began.

Those living with partners fared better, and of course, those with spacious, comfortable houses and gardens outside the city centre fared best of all. The lack of commute allowed them to spend more time in their comfortable homes. But they told me they had come to realise that their staff and loved ones living in different circumstances were struggling. Not only through lack of mentorship and training but also with their physical and mental health.

In my patient cohort it was the junior staff and trainees who suffered most of all, especially the new graduates. Many had just moved to London to start their careers and had gone straight into a highly stressful job where they were effectively flying solo. The regular Zoom calls allowed no room for the 'quick question' to keep them on the right track or to witness how their seniors spoke with clients. They had no respite at all. And many of them had contracted Covid in the first wave. I realised that lockdown damage was much greater and further reaching than I had imagined.

I could see that those told to stay inside and not meet anybody saw their physical and mental health decline. Frailty is like slow-setting glue. To stay as fit and healthy for as long as possible, you need to exercise both your mind and your body to delay the point at which this frailty becomes incompatible with life. But no risk was considered tolerable during lockdown, even the minor, almost negligible risk of going out for a walk, Tai Chi in the park or seeing a friend outside at a distance. During that beautiful spring and summer, the vulnerable were cooped up inside, lonely, and losing mental and physical function. Even two years later we were asked to see patients who became housebound during this period of shielding and who hadn't left their homes since.

As previously described, the co-dependent nature of our bodily systems means that if one is affected, all are. With less slack in the system, this is more problematic as you age. Losing muscle bulk can cause sarcopenia, resulting in an increased rate of immune system decay and a loss of anti-inflammatory protection, in addition to the more obvious reduction in functional ability. This discovery that muscle bulk is effectively a reservoir for the immune system has meant that, in recent years, regular strength training has been recommended as a form of immunotherapy.

To avoid cognitive decline, the recommendation is to prevent loneliness. Loneliness is a risk factor for depression, poor sleep, impaired thinking skills, increased use of health care, more medication and a higher rate of falls. Socialisation is important. The light of recognition that shines in the brain of an Alzheimer's sufferer grows dimmer over time, with that rate of change only slowed by repeated exposure. Even after this first lockdown, there were many reports from those whose loved ones no longer recognised them.

With an increase in frailty, we made our vulnerable more vulnerable still. If they were to be exposed to Covid, they would be less able to fight it. If they had a minor illness or surgery, they were less likely to survive it. The vulnerable were locked away and, tragically, many spent their remaining life in lockdown, with their lives both shortened by it and made miserable as a result of being cut off from their loved ones.

To maintain your physical function, you need to keep doing the activities you want to be able to continue to do. To manage the stairs, you keep using the stairs. To be able to go shopping, the balance, strength and cognitive skills required are best maintained by simply going to the shops. Functional fitness is activity specific: whilst some will have managed to stay strong by exercising indoors, many would not have managed to perform a broad enough range of activities to be able to function normally again by the time they were told it was safe to go outside.

The most shocking aspect of my clinical caseload was the sheer speed at which previously healthy, thriving individuals had become unwell. Those who had been able to work from home on full pay were those I had envied. Seeing these broken individuals was shocking. Those newspaper and social media articles on 'what to do during lockdown' looked even more like a cruel joke than before. None of these patients had learned to play the guitar or speak French, nor were they making sourdough or banana bread.

As September continued there was no doubt that cases and hospitalisations were rising. All who claimed it was over were clearly and demonstrably wrong. I was wrong. It was clear that there would be a second wave.

On 22 September the government called a press conference. Those who could work from home should go back to doing so, masks were back, and sports and gatherings were limited again. Businesses were to check people in using QR codes, and you would be allowed to take your mask off in a hospitality venue only when seated. The government anticipated that these restrictions would continue until March 2021.

Some thought these policies didn't go far enough. Campaigns had started for a two-week 'circuit breaker', a lockdown by another name. This would apparently be enough to keep case numbers down and stop the NHS from collapsing over the winter period. Vaccines were on the horizon, and these two weeks would buy us time until the vulnerable had been vaccinated. What I didn't understand was how reducing cases then, for two weeks only, would last until the depths of winter were over. It seemed more likely to push the peak into the worst possible time to have it.

I'd like to say that my concerns were solely for others at this stage, but that would be a lie. This was a disaster for me. My patient numbers had doubled in September to 30% of my normal caseload, giving me enough income to cover my fixed costs. After the work-from-home advice, I was instantly thrust into accruing debt at the rate of £2,000 a week again, despite still not taking dividends as pay. I also worried for those patients I had seen who had just emerged from the first lockdown. They would go back into their bedroom lives and be expected to work at full pelt for at least another six months. I was feeling pretty sorry for myself and all the businesses like mine that had seen a light at the end of the tunnel. There was at least as much again to come, and with our loans only designed to last until the end of September, there was a huge amount of panic, desperation and anger.

11 Reasons To Be Fearful: Part Two – The New Normal

Gyms and pools were still closed, so there were fewer opportunities to exercise. And we were only allowed to leave the house once a day. Working from home led to less physical activity. Not many were managing their ten thousand steps a day. Stress and boredom led to comfort eating. Many put on weight. Even children. Especially children. The level of restrictions we had, even at this point, was continuing to damage our health.

My fears now were that a large number of the unhealthy behaviours of restrictions had become the new default. Many would cease to notice what was missing from their former, healthier life, and their health would continue to deteriorate. For these people their unhealthy lifestyle and environment would conspire to cause a sensitised system, a hair trigger for a range of different illnesses. And by habituating to it, people's increased vulnerability to illness would go unnoticed.

The change from conscious to unconscious habitual behaviour is a little like changing from a manual to an automatic car. Or moving house and changing your commute. To begin with, you are conscious of the change and have to think about it, but eventually, you establish a new autopilot. It becomes mindless.

When looking at health in the individual, the apparent stimulus or risk factor for illness cannot be considered in isolation. An example is the pain of arthritis: whilst it is normal to have degenerative changes in joints beyond a certain age, most will not have symptoms. These changes do not cause the symptoms; they are a risk factor. This is why we 'treat the man, not the scan'. Chronic, low-grade, systemic inflammation is increasingly implicated as a reason for clinical risk factors to become symptomatic. There are activities and behaviours that create inflammation, and there are those that are anti-inflammatory. We need to ensure we do enough of the latter to stay well, but if our bodies tip into a more inflammatory state, illness will follow with the least provocation.

This is one of the many reasons why controls are so important in research: there is still much we do not understand about the function of asymptomatic individuals. Some can have the same measurable signs as those with symptoms, so great care has to be taken not to target interventions towards these measurable signs until you know, by comparing these signs with a group of matched asymptomatic controls, they are what is causing the problem rather than a harmless variation of normal. Seek and you shall find, but it may not be clinically relevant. Worse, the intervention designed to correct this errant finding may prove to be damaging, rather than just ineffective.

Occasionally chronic illnesses do subside, and people can return to their previous lives. This can happen when lifestyle triggers have been suppressed and dampened for a long period. This lets the mind and body desensitise, and a new default mechanism can be established, which becomes so well reinforced that intermittent stressors do not cause a relapse. A prolonged recuperation isn't available to most, unfortunately. For many with chronic illness, management includes permanent, significant lifestyle changes (for example, a change of occupation) just to keep symptoms manageable.

Insidious conditions (those without an obvious cause or which come on gradually) often result from a collection of different risk factors occurring simultaneously. Perhaps there is a genetic predisposition or a similarly unalterable risk, such as age. A recent illness leaving someone temporarily weaker. A bereavement, a deadline at work or a difficult relationship at home. A lack of control within one's life is a risk factor for many different illnesses. As is a poor diet or insufficient exercise. Poverty is often the largest trigger of all, as it has a disproportionate impact on all the above. Any of these risks and more can increase systemic inflammation and conspire to push you over the threshold into illness. You may identify one thing, one minor thing, but the truth is that for many their individual cocktail of risk ensured that whatever the trigger, theirs was an illness in waiting.

Good health is not something we should take for granted, but many do. Some assume that anyone not in good health is somehow to blame for it: certain chronic illnesses carry a stigma of self-inflicted injury. This is as untrue as it is unfair. Many environmental, social and genetic characteristics can prevent recovery, and many are not the fault of their owner.

The less control you have over the way you live your life and the fewer activities you enjoy that fill an emotional need, the more likely you are to indulge yourself in something unhealthy to make yourself feel better. Personal agency and the availability of joy should, in my opinion, be considered physiological needs, not luxuries. And if you have fewer possible sources of these, you are more likely to adopt an unhealthy activity to realise them. This is the core premise of the maintenance of good health for me: if you have control over the way you live your life, you are more likely to choose healthy behaviours to allow you to enjoy it more. Without enjoyment and fulfilment, there's little incentive to do anything other than something that brings short-term relaxation or pleasure.

In addition to a lack of understanding of the psychosocial determinants of ill health, there is a similar lack of understanding of behaviours that keep us well – social contact, physical touch, sex, singing and laughter. These activities, through activation of the parasympathetic nervous system, create an anti-inflammatory physiological response, allowing our pathways of relaxation and repair to counter the effects of stress on our minds and bodies, whether the sources of these stressors are physical or emotional. Although exercise has a temporarily stressful and inflammatory effect, the adaptive strength and fitness it confers not only make us stronger and fitter, but also produce a much longer-lasting, anti-inflammatory effect through increased muscle bulk. Muscle bulk is increasingly seen as an immune system reservoir and has an anti-inflammatory effect. It should be remembered that some stress, manageable stress, is good for us and essential to keep our physiology up to the tasks we impose upon it. But it has to be within our limits of tolerance, or it will injure us.

It interests me that only certain healthy activities are admired. Abstinence from the pleasure of a piece of cake or a glass of wine or making yourself exercise when you don't enjoy it are usually praised and celebrated, even when they are easy for some. Perhaps this is a direct result of Public Health messaging over the years. Not so praised is the ability to make and maintain friendships and avoid loneliness.

Loneliness is known to be bad for your health. There is a rich seam of information on the subject, and any literature search will turn up a horrifying list of health risks. Some medical papers estimate this risk to be equivalent to smoking fifteen cigarettes a day, way above the risks of obesity.

I wish there were a more general understanding of just how important the need for human contact is, even if some need it less than others. At the time I worried that this need, this physiological need for contact, had been overlooked and would become another risk factor for lockdown-related illnesses that would prove difficult to unwind.

For patients to recover from illness, environmental irritants need to be modified temporarily to allow the body to heal itself. Rest in the early stages, followed by a gradual reintroduction to normal life, may be enough for simple conditions to recover in the otherwise healthy person. But others will never be able to return fully to the life they led before. What is really fascinating is how illness can reveal a previous symptomatic pathway, the throbbing of a long-forgotten fracture during a viral illness, for example. Acute stress from whatever cause can seem to strip away the protective layers of new experience as the body tries to force you to slow down, allowing self-healing processes to kick in.

Another reason not to fire up the sympathetic system is that fear of a particular outcome can actually cause it to happen. I became interested in CBT partly to learn how to avoid catastrophisation through the use of nocebic language. Nocebo, the opposite of placebo, worsens outcomes. And telling people, for example, that their joint degeneration shown on an X-ray would result in pain and reduced function can become a self-fulfilling prophecy. The patient is scared to move and exercise, although this is the very approach that would help their pain and function. So, they have more pain and less function: clearly professionally irresponsible and best avoided.

In my cohort of patients, a small amount of pain can sometimes lead to an unusually strong emotional response. Those who have had severe pain and prolonged recoveries in the past can imagine this minor pain to be the first step on the pathway back to their previous level of pain and disability. They are understandably concerned. They seize up and stop moving naturally. Their worry fires up muscles into spasm, the joints move less, and the prior pain pathways are realised once again. My job is to assess the risk, of course, but also to encourage the patients to move in a way that will not elicit this response, avoiding the realisation of this self-fulfilling prophecy.

The first lecture of my CBT course has always stayed with me. If you want to avoid catastrophisation, you don't tell patients not to worry about relapsing into their previous pain state. The analogy used was to think of a flying pink elephant. If thinking of a flying pink elephant causes damage, the last thing you do is tell them to stop thinking of a flying pink elephant. The point was well made; solely by virtue of this discussion we could think of nothing other than flying pink elephants. Since this course I have sought to reassure by action instead and often by asking the patient to perform the movements that worry them. They are generally not reassured by my words; on the contrary, they may feel I disbelieve their symptoms. The best way clinically for me is to ask them to do it. Often when they do, it's a little sore. But on repetition it becomes less sore. (If, of course, it becomes more sore, I will change tack completely.)

Another worry was that by creating a new normal of the expectation of masks and social distancing, people would be fearful when these were removed. You cannot tell people repeatedly to be scared of maskless faces and then expect that fear to simply drop away. This fear, once inspired for long enough, would create neurophysiological changes perpetuating it, even when the risk is much lower. We had taught people to be fearful of a disease they could not see. Masks and social distancing were their protection against this threat. What would happen when they were removed? They would be fearful, and this fear may, on its own, cause or worsen illness. It would certainly reduce the immune system's ability to respond, given this is reliant on parasympathetic function.

Our parasympathetic system relies on the ability to relax, to allow the heart rate to drop, blood pressure to reduce, digestion to occur and all our subconscious systems to regulate and thrive. Much of its function is delivered through the vagus nerve. Activities supporting vagus nerve health include the following: physical touch, singing, laughter, socialisation and exercise. All of which, to a large extent, were banned by the mandating of restrictions during the pandemic. (Online interaction is not a replacement, as I shall describe later.)

The stress of the pandemic, regardless of what measures were implemented, had already created an ideal environment for the development of illness. Fear ramped up that signal. The choice of mandated restrictions banned many activities that could have helped prevent illness.

And by now this harmful way of life had become our normal.

12 The Circuit (Spirit) Breaker

I started October 2020 with a sense of foreboding. My business had tanked with the work-from-home order as I had predicted. Prominent commentators, who had only just started to discuss harms, stopped doing so. Restrictions came first, not resources. My husband would be away for work for five weeks from 12 October. And we were nowhere near back to normal.

Much debate was held between those who wanted to focus resources and restrictions on the vulnerable and those who insisted all transmissions should be suppressed. The Great Barrington Declaration espoused the former and the John Snow Memorandum, the latter. It seemed to me that your personal circumstances, whatever they were, would usually determine which approach you favoured. I knew my own bias: I couldn't bear the thought of another lockdown. But on 31 October the prime minister announced one; it would last four weeks and would start on 5 November.

On the first day of lockdown, inconsolable and alone, I ran to Parliament Square and wept, staring at the empty building. To rage at a parliament that wasn't there. Hadn't been there for months. An absent parliament cut off from the needs of the people it had been elected to represent.

The second wave of restrictions had plunged my emotional state back into black and white when I had just started seeing glimpses of colour. All hope for the future was lost. The feeling of desperation and frustration had me wondering how I had managed to fail quite so spectacularly. My life's work had been blown out as easily as a candle on a child's birthday cake. And with no remorse from those who extinguished it. They didn't even notice.

My husband was not allowed to come home for the weekends because of Covid. The children were back at school, masked and bubbled, with no sports fixtures, music concerts or extracurricular clubs because of Covid. School with all the fun taken out, but at least it allowed them to tread water. I had to work hard to keep my pain away from them. Cry only during the day. Be ready to take their troubles in the evening. Then once they went to bed, cry again or stare into space until collapsing into troubled, interrupted sleep.

I had been lucky in one sense: my landlord had agreed to waive the quarter's rent and the council had awarded me a £10,000 grant. But I was still losing £2,000 per week on zero pay. With the city deserted and companies changing their plans to stay away until at least February, the future was bleak. I know many businesses that closed in that time, never to reopen.

I had to hold it together for my family, for my staff and for me. I remembered previous conversations with my GP, who told me I'd be no good to my children if I were dead. The simplicity and truth of this hit me again. Much as I wanted and needed this to end, I had to figure out how to drop more gears and continue to wade slowly through treacle, avoiding panic and catastrophisation.

But it was so, so hard.

I found myself praying to go to sleep and wake again in March. It was to be a long winter of discontent, and the worst was yet to come.

13 'Tis the Season To Be 'Tiery'

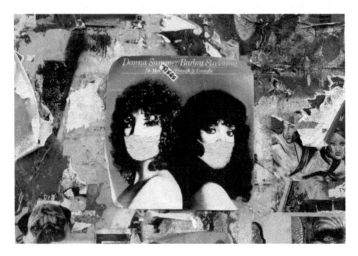

Since my late twenties I have been fortunate enough to have gone to the theatre for almost more weeks than I have not. At times I have seen more than I was expecting, from a naked Nicole Kidman in *The Blue Room*, by way of a naked James McAvoy in *Privates on Parade* and then to a naked Benedict Cumberbatch tumbling out of a fake placenta in *Frankenstein*, with all manner of displays of nudity in between.

I have seen the greatest stage actors of my generation in a wide range of different productions. I was privileged to see Helen McCrory in many productions before her untimely death in 2021. My first, *The Triumph of Love* at the Donmar Warehouse, I still remember clearly: when on stage, Helen's luminous quality and extraordinary embodiment of her character meant I only wanted to watch her and nobody else. This was as true of the last performance I saw, *Deep Blue Sea*, as it was of the first. I saw her *Medea*, as well as those starring Diana Rigg and Fiona Shaw. Too many great actors and great shows to mention; I have been very lucky. Of course, I've seen some terrible performances in some terrible shows too, but I shall leave those turns unstoned.

Another actor I have seen on many occasions is Simon Russell Beale. My favourite of his earlier performances was his Dr Pangloss in *Candide*. The overture had him striding in a clockwise direction on the Olivier revolve as it was turning the other way, with optimism beaming out of his brilliantly poised and posed persona as he strode apparently pointlessly on this stage's constructed treadmill. Another memorable turn by him was as Joseph Stalin in *Collaborators* where he expertly lured Alex Jennings' Bulgakov into signing the orders for the Great Purge. If pressed I think my favourite performance of his would be in *The Lehman Trilogy*, the story of three immigrant brothers founding an investment firm. Not as dry as it sounds. He and the other two actors, Ben Miles and Adam Godley, played all the parts; it was extraordinarily staged and inspiringly directed by Sam Mendes. At one point Simon Russell Beale transformed convincingly from a strict, observant, serious grandfather into a spoilt, coquettish granddaughter with the merest twirl of his hand.

One of my favourite aspects of attending the theatre is the shared audience experience. You get a sense of it even when this is negative rather than positive. In a less successful production people start to fidget. They look around and raise their usually English, middle-class eyebrows to show disapproval. If it's really bad, people start to mutter. A Mexican wave of barely suppressed displeasure rolls through the audience. If it's really, really bad, the unmistakable tones of 'oh, for goodness' sake' will surely emanate from some disgruntled witness.

But when it is good, nobody moves. This happens rarely, but when it does it is magical. Instead of a chorus of disharmony, it's as if everyone breathes as one. Nobody shifts to relieve a numb bottom or a stiff back. Knees stay uncrossed, unsore and unnoticed. Of course, there may be one idiot with a bag of Werther's Originals, slowly unwrapping one sweet after another, but they can be dealt with. When watching *The Lehman Trilogy*, for example, the offender behind was unmoved by the muttering of the gentleman to my right. I sat bolt upright and leaned forwards a bit. At the next pause she leaned towards me and tapped me on the shoulder. 'Could you please sit back in your seat?' she asked. 'Only if you stop eating your boiled sweets,' I replied. The elderly gentleman beside me responded with what I can only describe as a guffaw and then, 'Oh, well done!' He told me he would relocate during the interval just in case, but it did feel like I'd scored a particularly British kind of victory.

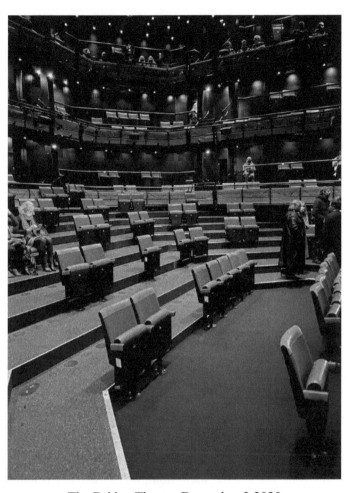

The Bridge Theatre December 3 2020

I had booked to see *A Christmas Carol* with Simon Russell Beale as Scrooge on 3 December 2020. Luckily for us, it was the day after England emerged from the second coronavirus lockdown, and the performance could go ahead: under the tier system, London was in Tier Two, meaning that most businesses could open but with very strict Covid guidelines in place. My daughter and I were very much looking forward to it. We had seen the joyous Old Vic interpretation a couple of years previously with Rhys Ifans as Scrooge; mince pies and clementines were handed out on arrival, and the finale was punctuated by the cascade of huge plastic turkeys and various Christmas foods via cloth chutes from the Grand Circle. The Bridge's 2020 version was to be very different.

When theatres reopened they tried to reduce costs and the risk of cancellation by having small casts (often monologues), virtually no sets and no intervals. The bars were shut to avoid mingling and crowding. When we arrived at the Bridge Theatre we were checked at the door and told to keep our masks on and keep our distance. Ushered through to the auditorium, we saw that two rows of seats out of every three had been completely removed; the remaining batches of one to six seats had been grouped by household bookings, as per Covid regulations. We nodded to our friends sitting three metres or so away and sat down.

This version of the play had three people playing all the parts and almost nothing on stage: only two trunks with costume changes and a few boxes in the corner. One wall across the middle with a door for entrances and exits. It was a more traditional, dark interpretation of the book too, and I will always remember Simon Russell Beale mouthing 'thank you for coming' at the curtain call.

Theatres made what they could of it, but it was a soulless experience completely lacking in atmosphere. So tough for the performers: grateful to be performing at all but performing to a largely empty room. For me it seemed a slightly out-of-body experience, watching the audience as much as the stage, wondering how and when I had walked through the door to this half-familiar, half-dystopian parallel world.

Bars and pubs could open too, but only if serving a 'substantial meal'. When pressed, a government representative suggested a Scotch egg would suffice. How ridiculous! What possible purpose could this serve? Parody after parody appeared on social media, and the substantial meal became an effective beer tax. For our local this was vegetable soup. It was completely disgusting. But the beer was, as always, fabulous. As was the welcome. Our lovely publican had also paid for scaffolding and heaters to make it warm enough to sit outside. With the burble and buzz of a full, albeit seated, grateful pub, he was in fine form.

But sadly for the businesses, London was placed into Tier Three at midnight on 15 December. They hadn't even been open for two weeks. All that planning, all that cost, all the expensive risk assessments and extra precautions had been for nothing.

The Kent variant of Covid, subsequently known as Alpha, had started to spread rapidly in London. In schools the sixth formers seemed to get it first, and this time, unlike the original variant, it spread to the younger years. My daughter's senior school had, following a discussion with Public Health England, reverted to online schooling for the last week of term, but my younger daughter's school stayed open. It was curious: my WhatsApp parent groups reported that in my older daughter's class of twenty-four children, there were six confirmed cases the week before the school closed. In my younger daughter's junior school there were apparently none. (We were informed by email each time there was a case, and there had only been one family affected much earlier on in the term just after they returned from their summer holiday.)

We were due to leave for a holiday on 20 December; by lunchtime on 19 December the bags were packed and in the hall. It was clear by then that it would be a grim winter, but I hoped the holiday would give us some respite and help us get through the next bit. Sadly for us, the prime minister, Boris Johnson, called a press conference for 4 pm on 19 December. An hour before check-in our holiday disappeared as London was plunged into a new tier: Tier Four. In reality it was lockdown by another name: this tier had the same restrictions as Lockdown Two. And this time the schools had closed for the Christmas break. So, although the official lockdown started later when all areas of England were assigned Tier Four, for us it started at midnight on 19 December.

And it would last longer than the first. Much, much longer.

14 The Bleak Midwinter

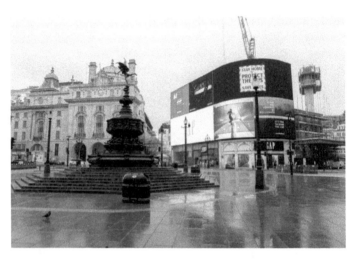

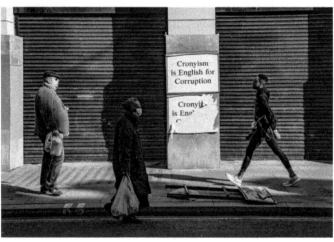

The third lockdown started officially on 6 January. Schools reopened for one day before closing again, despite the promise they would be 'last to close and first to open'. The build-up to this was fraught and angry on both sides. I dreaded how awful the next couple of months would be. I just hoped it would be less bad than I anticipated, that any damage would be reversible and that we'd be allowed to recover at the end of it without the threat of further closures.

What I didn't understand was why the well-run system administered by Public Health England had been shut down in favour of an indiscriminate, nationwide closure. We had been geared up to start twice-weekly lateral flow testing after an initial two tests taken closely together. This aimed to prevent those who were infectious from returning to senior school and to limit outbreaks going forwards. I also thought that such a large outbreak would prevent reinfection, or at least prevent rapid reinfection. I certainly saw no reason at all for my younger daughter's school to close, given there had been no outbreaks at all.

Sadly, what took weeks to have an emotional effect in Lockdown One took only days in Lockdown Three. It was the depths of winter with the dark and dreich outside as a worthy background to our despair. But the weather wasn't the main reason for the speed of the deterioration. The damage from Lockdown One had simply been too great to undo in so short a time. The only possibility of recovery was to make life bigger around the damage, but the trigger had been pulled without the increased experience to act as a buffer. The wound had not yet healed. The misery memory was swiftly realised.

Children had nothing to offset the effects of this new school closure. They couldn't meet a friend unless they could travel alone and on foot (under-fives could be accompanied). Only one person from two different households could meet outside. And not to play, only to walk or run.

Playgrounds were allowed to remain open this time, but many shut anyway. As playgrounds were the only legal place for children to play outside their own homes, they became popular and too crowded for zealous local councils to tolerate.

Playing outside anywhere else, even in the park, was forbidden. Memorably, two brothers aged six and eight were sent home by the police for building a snowman in the park. Sent home to build one in the garden they didn't have.

Adults were allowed to exercise outdoors in pairs. But children don't get their exercise by running and chatting with a friend two metres apart, masked and jogging. They exercise through play.

Perhaps for families living in a rural environment with a garden and more than one child, the children were shielded from the worst effects. Some may have appeared to thrive. At the time. But thriving in solitude may be more concerning than suffering: how are they to learn to have satisfying relationships as adults if they don't figure it out as children during those critical periods of emotional development?

Some parents enjoyed having their children at home and spending more time with them. But not all could find that time, of course: this luxury would only apply to those who didn't have to work.

Perhaps if the children were small and the parents were available, they managed not too badly. Children are entirely dependent on adults to begin with, and the passageway to adulthood is a steady disengagement from dependency. Those with small children were tearing their hair out, but the children may have fared better since they had more of what they needed. But not those at nursery, who were learning to communicate with masked carers and missing the opportunity to hardwire human attachment into their rapidly developing brains. And, of course, they were losing out on the opportunity to mirror smiles, observe the articulation of language and mimic both so that they could witness, learn, repeat and achieve that catalyst for human connection.

Those who had shielded through the summer were shielding again. This time, with ice on the roads and a higher risk of falling, it was more difficult to encourage our frail citizens to keep exercising. The temptation to hibernate was high, and many were understandably scared to venture outside because of Covid too, even after their vaccination. At my practice we saw many people who never recovered their mobility after this period. It was a shame this wasn't recognised more as a risk at the time, as there was a great deal we could have done to prevent it or minimise the deterioration if we had seen the patients soon enough.

One piece of music became my soundtrack to this dreadful, dreadful time. 'E lucevan le stelle', a romantic aria from the opera *Tosca*, is sung by Tosca's lover, Cavaradossi, as he attempts to describe the joy she brought to him in a love letter before his death.

My daughter had just started learning the clarinet part. This melody, this beautiful melody of misery, was an appropriate companion for the darkness outside our homes and inside our hearts. Each time she played it, its tragic legato phrasing penetrated the small part of me still able to feel. The relentlessness of its course struck me like a slowly turning, inevitable but unstoppable corkscrew. The numbness would temporarily abate, forcing me to acknowledge just how awful this was, how there seemed no prospect of an end to it.

Unlike the first lockdown we were allowed to see patients face to face, so I continued commuting to my practice twice a week. Without the office workers I had very little to do, but it felt good to be able to leave the house and go in, even if it was to see only one patient and say hello to my colleagues.

In Lockdown One I looked up and around me at the emptiness of the West End and my local Pimlico neighbourhood. This time I was struck by the lifeless carcass of the City. Without the modernity of its occupants, the sense of history became more arresting and more impressive. Much of this area burned down in the Great Fire of London, to be reimagined by the architect Sir Christopher Wren and to be painstakingly restored after the Blitz. On leaving Mansion House tube station on my commute, I always walk up Bow Lane – a narrow, cobbled street lined with small shops on both sides. I take time to look left at the junction with Watling Street to see St Paul's Cathedral, which in January 2021 was cast in a surprising orange glow by the late dawns of winter.

Just before the top of Bow Lane, I turn left into the churchyard of St Mary-le-Bow. Originally a Saxon church, St Mary-le-Bow is the home of the famous Bow Bells: you can call yourself a Cockney only if born within listening distance. Turning left on Cheapside, I pass Bread Street and Milk Street and turn right on Wood Street to walk up to the Barbican complex.

As you approach London Wall, there are escalators up to the podium level where you meet the southernmost border of the Barbican Estate. After being heavily bombed in the Second World War, the parish of Cripplegate was redesigned as a residential community in the brutalist style and built in the 1960s. (St Giles was the patron saint of the lame, thus Cripplegate was his parish.)

Before I moved into the Barbican, it occupied an empty space between the City and Clerkenwell in my mental map of central London. I had stumbled into it once or twice, got lost and vowed never to darken its doors again. I thought it was extremely ugly and very confusing. As someone with no sense of direction, I found it disorientating and alienating, even without the imposing nature of its concrete structure.

Now I think it's beautiful. Everything works. You can walk from one side to the other using the second-floor walkways without crossing a single road. Cars live in the basement car parks, not on the street. The buildings are dotted around the Barbican Lake. With the steadily increasing height of buildings all around, it appears like a surprise oasis of calm amidst the cacophony of commerce.

The older walkways hug the straight lines of each building like gutters; newer additions are rivers snaking around the modern office blocks and derelict parts of the old city wall. Beautifully planned, they open out intermittently to reveal a small patch of grass or a welcome bench.

It is a community. Business premises in the Barbican include a kindergarten, a school, an arts centre, a college and practices like mine. Residents feel proud and privileged to live there and are defensive of its aesthetic reputation. It is certainly a taste I have ended up acquiring.

My route to work passes many shops, from those selling expensive city clothes and shoes to the ubiquitous coffee and vaping shops. There are chemists, food stores and a Daunt Books shop too. With an absence of commuters into the City, every single one of them closed (even the Greggs on Cheapside) except for one coffee shop – Black Sheep Coffee on Wood Street. On the two days a week I went in, I was sure to buy something even if I didn't want it, and I was very sad when it, too, closed at the end of January.

15 The Nightingale

In mid-December the NHS bank had approached me to see if I would be willing to train and work as a vaccinator. After a repeat of the extraordinary number of forms for Test and Trace, another interview, a DBS criminal records check and the additional requirement of the records of my medical screening and vaccinations, I was offered the work. I would be working at Chelsea and Westminster Hospital.

Whilst waiting for the job to begin, I was contacted again and asked if I would be able to work at the Nightingale Hospital at the ExCel exhibition centre in east London instead. This meant another job application, verification of documents and a further DBS criminal records check. This time the recruitment came through an agency: I would not be employed but engaged on a zero-hours contract. And this time I'd be working as a physiotherapist.

The Nightingale hospitals had been set up in the first wave as overflow intensive care units for those who were acutely and severely ill. The ExCel exhibition centre was converted into a hospital in an astonishing nine days: it had five hundred fully fitted beds with oxygen and ventilators, with the capacity to increase to four thousand beds.

In the end only fifty-four patients were treated there in the first wave. It was lucky that the demand was less than anticipated, not only because it meant there were fewer ill people, but also because there were apparently not enough specialised staff to run these facilities. (I remember in the first wave that the only volunteers who were offered work were trained ITU (intensive therapy unit) staff. Those of us working in different specialties were not used, as far as I know.)

This time the Nightingale would be used as a 'step-down' facility for those who were not acutely medically unwell but lacked the physical independence to be discharged back to their homes. It would be GP led with a team of occupational therapists, physiotherapists and social service liaison staff to physically rehabilitate, organise any increased care or equipment and ensure the patients were capable of returning home. In part we would help alleviate the log jam caused by the lack of social care: some of the patients we treated were those often referred to as 'bed blockers'.

The induction process, though admin-heavy and a repeat of my previous experiences, was done at pace. I had my first phone call on Wednesday 6 January and started my induction on Saturday, three days later.

On the first day of my induction, Saturday 9 January, the UK had the most deaths in a day since the start of the pandemic. But I wasn't scared of catching Covid; I was more nervous about being useful. It wouldn't be complicated work but would be a completely different demographic from what I was used to, with much more pain and disability. Although the agency offered me a different pay band, I signed on as a band five, equivalent to a new graduate.

When I arrived at Custom House station, I was aware of someone close behind as I gingerly negotiated the frozen ground. A GP who had set up the rehabilitation wards, working every day since Boxing Day. He was hoping to have a day off soon, and I wished him well.

On reaching the entrance there was a long queue of people signing in and picking up temporary passes; once done, we were directed to the induction room. This was huge, like an aircraft hangar: stripped to bare white walls and occupied only by spaced-out chairs and a massive screen. A few people knew each other ('you at the Cromwell too?') and tried to communicate across the social distance and the muffling effect of masks, but most sat quietly, reading or looking at their phones. Some had been here in the first wave when ITU patients were admitted. They were 'old hands'. The general feeling was that this field hospital was better planned, more comfortable and more spacious. This time they could switch off the overhead lights so that patients could sleep. Most attendees had NHS jobs during the week and would only be working weekends for overtime. My weekday cohort of workers consisted mainly of private practitioners. Our managers were NHS secondees, who knew the process and knew the complex admin system within which we were to work.

Then we had a tour; we were shown where to pick up our scrubs and where we were to change clothes. Through to a common anteroom where we would re-sanitise and display our roles by sticking differently coloured electrical tape on our shoulders. Then on to the ward itself. I was struck by people sitting on floors in the corridors, regularly spaced and scrubbing. Scrubbing what? I wasn't sure; it looked as if they were sealing and smoothing gaps between the strips of lino. On to the ward itself, where carpenters were redrilling the toilet door hinges to open outwards rather than inwards. The reassuring presence of army personnel in fatigues, with a wide stance and folded arms, exuded competence, composure and reliability.

A lot of induction followed: procedural training on how to use Rio (the NHS software) – slowly, repetitively and painfully, and basic life-support training. No mouth-to-mouth resuscitation was allowed either in or out of training, owing to the risk of Covid transmission. No chest compressions were to be performed without full PPE, since this aerosol-generating procedure would make the surgical mask ineffective. Defibrillator first, whilst someone gowns up. Still a lot of questions.

Two days later my first weekday commute to the Nightingale was an eye-opener. This was not the quiet District Line experience into the City. This time I took the Jubilee Line, changing to the DLR (Docklands Light Railway) at Canning Town. Canning Town was packed full of people changing trains. The DLR carriages were crammed with people who were shown by statistics to be the most vulnerable to Covid, namely those categorised by the ONS (Office for National Statistics) as working in 'low-skilled elementary occupations' such as construction and security. All on their way to work, and all unprotected by lockdown. Once again I wondered if those who talked of reducing community transmission to protect the vulnerable had any idea of this reality. Here were the vulnerable crammed into carriages on their way to their essential jobs.

As I arrived on the ward, the chief executive officer was thanking everyone and outlining the plan for reopening. The army personnel present at the induction were still scattered about, sleeves rolled up, looking busy and efficient. A lieutenant colonel spoke after the CEO, describing briefly but clearly how the army had helped, finishing up with a cheery 'let's get to work'. Given my prior employment in a military hospital, I found their presence very reassuring. My army colleagues had been efficient, thorough, speedy and unflappable.

After the opening team talk, we were sent off in different directions for various types of on-the-job training, including how to perform and report our twice-weekly lateral flow tests. At that time these were a novelty, though they were quickly to become a way of life. We were also offered a Covid vaccination. Conveniently, an enormous vaccination centre had been set up at the other end of the ExCel building. This had undergone a soft opening the day before, but today was the first attempt to get as many through as possible. We stood in line in our white scrubs in a snaking line of the over-eighties. All were waiting patiently, some in wheelchairs, some leaning precariously on a stick or a pair of crutches. Volunteers scurried around placing chairs at equal distances but realised in the process that we needed more wheelchairs. Why? Because you can't just move to a different chair; they needed to be wiped down between occupants.

Despite this, nobody grumbled. It was a remarkably positive and optimistic experience, slightly reminiscent of airport check-in. But instead of people going on holiday, these were the very old – much closer to the end of their lives than the beginning. They wanted to live. It made me proud to be British; we had prioritised those who were most at risk from Covid, not those with the most wealth or influence.

Each morning would start with a multidisciplinary meeting followed by one on rehabilitation. Patients were listed on a whiteboard with targets and goals; these were discussed, and we were assigned our caseload.

On the ward the patients were the very old, usually with several comorbidities. Different illnesses had put them in hospital, but many had been deteriorating steadily beforehand and were too frail to return to their previous level of independence. These comorbidities ranged from heart problems, strokes, Parkinsonism, cancer and broken hips, amongst others.

They were a joy to work with. When I first graduated I found it particularly difficult to make conversation with elderly patients, but this time around it was different. At fifty years old I saw other people's mums and dads, their sisters and brothers, and their children. Instead of their medical condition, I saw their stories, their lives and their loves. We would discuss these whilst I helped them to walk, wash, eat or move around more easily.

My best moment at the Nightingale came out of my idle chatter – attempts to connect with my patients as human beings. I had the early shift, so I would help them gain independence when eating breakfast. They had toast with butter, honey or jam, but so many of them were upset about the absence of marmalade. I didn't understand this distress, so I asked one old lady (ninety-nine years old with gloriously long, beautiful white hair) to explain it.

Apparently, during the Second World War they couldn't get hold of marmalade. When it finally reappeared, it indicated that the war was over. It held a great deal of emotion for them, and its absence had an extraordinarily adverse effect on their state of mind. I spoke to my line manager about this and asked if I would be allowed to bring in some individual sachets. Even better – she asked the caterers to put some on order. The elderly patients were all smiles and full of happy chatter after their marmalade arrived. Extraordinary. But very, very gratifying to be able to do something quite so simple to bring them a little joy.

On the other face of the dial, I treated someone who wasn't improving despite having been in hospital for three weeks. He wasn't very interested in moving around; he just wanted to go home. However much we encouraged him, he often refused to try to stand up. In the end that was his choice, so we arranged the maximum level of care for him and complied with his wishes. I told him excitedly about arranging for marmalade to come with his toast in the morning. 'I can't stand marmalade,' he said.

∞

Coming from the private sector and not having worked in the NHS for twenty-five years, I was used to a very different way of working. My aim in private practice is to minimise administration time so that I can spend more time with patients. I find admin exceptionally dull; I only get paid for the time I am with patients, and being with patients is what I find most rewarding. So, I have designed our day-to-day notes to be quick to access and record, whilst being GDPR (General Data Protection Regulation) compliant and secure to an EU standard. I have mechanised measuring and auditing as much as possible, and all our systems talk to each other.

My practice management system is set up to create data on demand through a series of templates and merge fields that I have designed for my company's and my clients' specific needs. With large corporate contracts I provide a great deal of data: how many treatments per case, what the outcomes are and which departments have a specific issue with particular areas of complaint, for example. But this is all programmed to draw through and be analysed on demand.

I don't know if the administrative burden was due to the temporary nature of the Nightingale or if it is embedded within the NHS. What I read from the newspapers and have heard from my NHS colleagues suggests the latter. But I know it was arduous. The last time I'd worked in the NHS, we used a notes trolley with paper notes: everything was recorded there, and it didn't take long to do. This time we would have to find a spare computer, insert our Rio card and then wade through four different, torturously slow security windows to log in. We would then find the patient's record, enter the information in three different parts of the patient's notes and log out again. We were supposed to log in and out between every patient so that the time stamp would be correct. This process would take at least fifteen minutes.

It all took so long. I may have spent only five minutes with the patient, taking them to the loo or for a short walk, but I then had to spend much more time than that to record the event. A few of us ended up seeing patient after patient, jotting down a few notes on a piece of paper as we went along, then finding a computer on an empty ward to record everything at the end of the morning and then again at the end of the day. For physio it was less critical to record in real time, as opposed to the administration of drugs, and I probably tripled the amount of time I spent with the patients by doing it this way. Before using this system, I would be surprised if I spent more than one hour of my eight-hour shift with patients, even after I'd completed the training.

The discharge process was painfully long and complicated. The discharge manager would start at 4 pm, and if any of the pieces of paper were missing, the patient couldn't go home. I could have understood this if it were important information, but large sections of these reports seemed to focus on standardised reporting that was irrelevant to the individual patient. But it all had to be there. My NHS colleagues, seemingly used to this process, would stay without pay late into the evening to complete these tasks, but I wondered if these reports would ever be read.

A less obvious problem about entering a new environment with a mask-wearing mandate is that I'd never met the people I was working with before. The only people at the hospital not wearing a mask at all times were the patients. So, the way of recognising people altered. How tall were they? How did they hold themselves? The only part of their face you could see was their eyes.

I had a meeting with the person running the ward, my senior manager. The only person sitting in the office turned around as I approached. I saw that she wasn't wearing a mask and kept my distance. 'Can you tell me where to find X?' I asked. 'That's me!' she said, looking at me oddly. I hadn't recognised her. Her mask had become part of her face, without it she didn't look the same person. Particularly curious, since she wore her own clothes, not scrubs, which were very stylish and distinctive. I took all this in, recognised the hair too and felt extremely foolish. 'You look completely different with your mask off!' I spluttered. Except, of course, bar a small part of her overall appearance, she looked exactly the same. And weirdly, when she put the mask back on, I relaxed, as my brain was finally satisfied that I was actually speaking to the right person.

We had a continuous small trickle of patients starting two or three days after the hospital opened. After a couple of weeks, they loosened the admission criteria to try to encourage more referrals, but it was never busy. And unlike the first wave, this wasn't due to a lack of staff – perhaps the referral process was as complex as the discharge process and acted as a disincentive. I also heard the suggestion of resentment from other parts of the NHS: there was a lot of focus on the Nightingale hospitals, and they felt it was a 'Cinderella' service, taking attention away from their more pressurised institutions. Perhaps they were unwilling to refer patients to us.

Whatever the reason, the second iteration of the Nightingale hospital in London treated fewer than one hundred patients and closed in April 2021. I worked there for five weeks before they decided to start winding it down, texting me during my February half-term break to let me know my services were no longer required.

The Nightingale gave me purpose. I would arrive home, physically tired but mentally rested. I slept very, very well. I had camaraderie, the knowledge I had done something useful, close contact with a range of people, and the emotional reward of connecting with patients and helping them regain their independence.

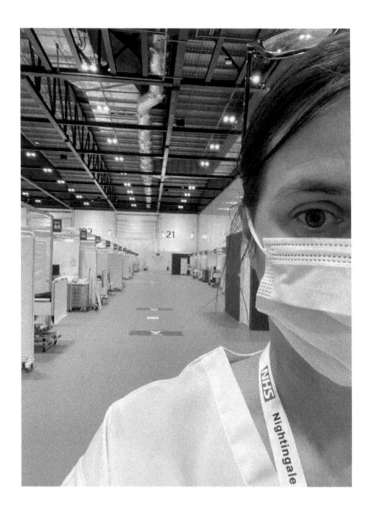

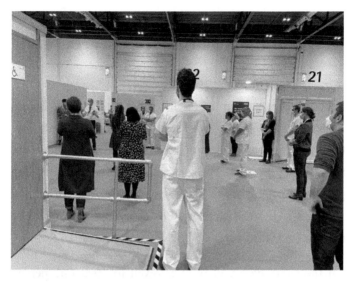
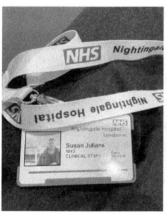
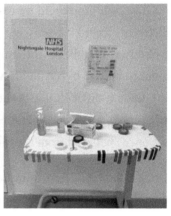

16 Unintended Consequences

Schools reopened on 8 March for the three weeks before Easter. Still bubbles, masks, twice-weekly lateral flow testing for secondary schools and isolation of contacts. But at least they opened. The government outlined a four-step pathway to come out of lockdown. We were promised that although individual steps may be delayed, there would be no step backwards.

On the same date you were allowed to meet one person outside your household for exercise. I had many walks with different friends discussing just how much worse this lockdown had been for our children, how much more quickly they suffered and how deeply. One friend tells me she finds it difficult now to go to the same spot in the park where we walked several times. Seeing the bandstand where we once sheltered from the rain is just too upsetting for her.

Once I had recovered from Long Covid, I continued to run outside through the darkest of times and the darkest of lockdown months. I love the freedom of running, the meditation of it. The way your footfall matches your heart rate. The feeling when your reservoirs of muscle glycogen are depleted and anaerobic capacity exhausted. The ability to continue running requires the metabolism of stored carbohydrate and fat. The ability to keep going and your running speed are dictated by the rate of oxygen delivery and take-up, both for combustion and the generation of kinetic energy.

Keen runners know this feeling as 'the zone'. Your body feels like a well-oiled machine, and you achieve the sensation of complete calm. When you hit this point, it feels like you can run forever. It's intoxicating. Your body is working in balance, and these co-dependent systems are working together harmoniously. If you like listening to music, finding the perfect tempo to fit with this rate enhances the sense of holistic completeness to an almost trance-like state.

Being able to return to running when my body finally cleared the virus was a huge relief. During this time, this selfish running time, I could focus on myself. I could escape from my responsibilities, achieve calm and peace away from the noise, and stabilise my mood for a complete and cathartic release. I would find the music that suited my mood, playing songs on a loop in the same way I did as a teenager. The same music too. Memories of my adolescent angst yielded a multitude of musical references.

But I really, really struggled to run whilst wearing a mask.

Various campaigners had encouraged universal mask-wearing from an early stage. Whilst this seemed logical when transmission was thought to be primarily through droplets, I couldn't understand how cloth masks could block something airborne, particularly if the viral particles were many times smaller than the weave of the cloth (as they turned out to be). But this advocacy for cloth masks carried a great deal of weight. From the start of the second wave, people walking with their one allotted friend would do so two metres apart widthways, leaving you nowhere to go but through the middle or into the path of oncoming traffic.

I remembered the amount of protection we needed at the Nightingale if we were to attempt life support or treat a Covid-positive patient: two surgical masks, a visor, gloves and a disposable gown covering your arms from the wrist and the rest of your body to the knee. And that was only until we had the chance to be fit tested for better masks. (The Nightingale wasn't even supposed to be open for active Covid cases.) Surely, the only thing they could recommend by now was the use of surgical masking, or even fit-tested masks? Even more nonsensical, it seemed, since a SAGE (Scientific Advisory Group for Emergencies) paper on outside transmission published in December 2020 had found this risk to be so small as to be almost negligible.

Before that paper emerged, my technique to reduce transmission risk had been to hold my breath if I had to pass someone at close distance. And if I wasn't running between two people, to turn away from whoever I was passing. I tried running with a surgical mask, having it high enough to be held down by my glasses and with the straps adjusted to minimise gaps. But I couldn't make it work. Not only did my glasses steam up, but because I had adjusted the fit, the mask would suck in and out of my mouth and nose, making it impossible to breathe properly.

My stubbornness meant I was unwilling to do something as seemingly pointless as wearing a cloth mask. It seemed its only effect would be to dehumanise, prevent human connection and communication, and perpetrate a lie for the sake of virtue collectivism.

Eventually, the stares of disapproval became too much. I stopped running completely. How was it to be relaxing and meditative when you're repeatedly being glared at? And with the mask restricting my breathing, the 'zone' I aspired to would have become an uncomfortable, fast and gasping walk at best.

ॐ

I had been asked again if I would be willing to train as a vaccinator. More forms and another interview followed. I attended a day of training on 19 March in a building just off Soho Square. This building reminded me of an old school with peeling paint, rattling sash windows and an incongruous, enormous picture of a young Princess Margaret hung badly on the wall.

The training was excellent – very efficient and comprehensive. There were around eight of us attending. At the end of the training, we were told we would be contacted the following Monday to book and plan our first shifts.

That contact never came. I emailed three or four times but received no response. As my work had started to pick up, I decided to leave it there and not pursue any further offers of work. Just as well, as none came.

On 29 March the second part of Step One of the government's roadmap out of lockdown commenced – two households were allowed to meet outside.

Before this step took effect, a young woman called Sarah Everard disappeared from Clapham Common. For so many women this was almost like a personal loss. Many of us thought of the times we had been vulnerable and managed to get away. The response also reminded me of the collective response to the death of Diana, Princess of Wales.

On both occasions the shock was a lightning rod for all our losses. And in Diana's case, there had been crowds and crowds of distressed, weeping mourners at Buckingham Palace every day. Thousands of bunches of flowers and dedications spread well into The Mall for weeks afterwards. She was 'the people's princess', said Prime Minister Tony Blair. But did we really care about the person, or were we distressed by the thought of death in one so young, who we assumed would be a presence throughout our lives? Did it remind us we were all going to die one day?

Despite the coronavirus regulations, there was to be a vigil for Sarah Everard around the Clapham Common bandstand on Saturday night. The family asked people not to go. They wanted to remember and grieve their loved one silently, privately and with dignity. An alternative was mooted: let us all light a candle on our doorsteps in a moment of peace. Let's wonder how we can make the world a better place. The victim was a gentle, generous soul – let us find something appropriate. When the family made this plea, I stayed home. I lit a candle, placed it on the doorstep and sat watching the flickering flame for a while with my older daughter.

Sadly, the vigil ended up in controversy with several women arrested and the police accused of heavy-handedness. I felt terribly sad for the family – this was the opposite of what they had wanted.

Instead, I ran to the bandstand early the next day on Mothering Sunday. All the trampled flowers had been removed. People had brought their Mother's Day flowers to lay down in silent tribute. Men, women, children. The very young and the very old. It was extraordinarily moving and humbling.

What this whole episode had shown though, was how coronavirus regulations could be used opportunistically by those who would cause us harm, particularly those who wanted to target the vulnerable. Sarah Everard thought she was being arrested. Instead, the police officer abducted her and later raped and killed her. (He has since been convicted of this crime.) The response to this was less than impressive: women were advised to stay home at night. They were told that if they didn't trust a police officer, they should flag down a bus instead. This came not from Twitter, but from senior police officers in statements to the press.

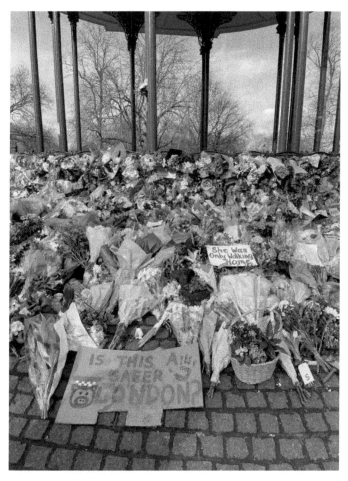

Vigil for Sarah Everard, Clapham Common March 14 2021

17 The Resistance To Reopening

The steps out of lockdown continued.

Step Two beginning on 12 April was a bigger change: leisure, hospitality and retail reopened with some restrictions. Hospitality was limited to table service outside, but at least the farce of a 'substantial meal' and curfews had been abandoned. The sun shone, it was the Easter holidays, and we took full advantage. Chinatown reopened with Gerrard Street covered in outside tables. On one occasion we visited Chinatown on the same day as a 'no questions asked' travelling vaccination centre, which attracted an enormous queue of local workers and residents.

Panton Street, home of Korean fried chicken, became my children's favourite spot. On our first visit we were the only ones there, with just one of the restaurants open. It was a joy to see it become fuller and fuller each time we walked past on the way into town.

It felt like we were slowly emerging from a very dark tunnel.

Many didn't feel that way, and articles started to appear in the mainstream press discussing the pros and cons of reopening. The vulnerable had been offered two vaccines, or would soon be, so I didn't understand why people still felt that restrictions and their associated harms were justified. I'd thought the deal was that restrictions would continue until all the vulnerable had been offered the opportunity to be vaccinated. From my biased and inexpert position, that was the social contract: those damaged by the restrictions would be allowed to resume their lives once modern science had done as much as it could to help those particularly vulnerable to the infection.

But even after the vaccine became available, some were still vulnerable to Covid. They had managed to avoid catching it for a year, so why would the restrictions change? Their vulnerability had not. The vaccines on their own had not managed to stamp out the virus completely. If restrictions were relaxed, some would be exposed.

I don't know if these individuals had been misled by the arrival of the vaccine, but I certainly had been. I had thought that with a 95% lower chance of contracting Covid, this would be enough to avoid future waves, and those who were unable to have the vaccine would be protected by this wall of immunity. Vaccines would allow us to attain the elusive herd immunity, and life could resume without the risk of large epidemic waves. But this was not the position we found ourselves in, at least not yet. Perhaps this would be possible when the younger years had access to the vaccine, as some suggested. The vaccine rollout continued at pace and started to extend into younger and younger age groups.

With Step Three on the roadmap out of lockdown, children were finally allowed to meet their friends inside on 17 May.

My daughter's birthday could be a sleepover. We were allowed to travel to see my mum for the first time in a year and a half. (Overnight stays were forbidden before Step Three, and she had shielded through the summer of 2020.) Finally, she cuddled her grandchildren again.

Step Three also allowed indoor hospitality venues to reopen – with masks on and Covid checks at the door – but they were open. We started visiting our old haunts again and had our first trip back to the theatre to see a revival of the play *Constellations* at the Vaudeville Theatre.

The Vaudeville Theatre is a slightly cramped, typically Victorian theatre on the Strand. Instead of taking out the seats (as the Bridge Theatre did back in December 2020), they simply had a 'social distancing' laminated sign stuck on the back of the ones that lay empty. There were two seats free on either side between each group booking, and one seat free in front and behind. The bar was closed.

I very much enjoyed it at the time, although it feels odd to look back on it. I wondered again how it was for the actors; with the audience so separated, it didn't feel like a collective experience. I would have loved to find out how it was for Zoë Wanamaker and Peter Capaldi, up there in a two-handed play with virtually no set. The audience showed its appreciation for sure; for a long time after theatres reopened, it seemed that each performance was celebrated with a standing ovation. But still, one of the joys of being in an audience for me is that sense of shared occasion, a shared experience with strangers. A roomful of people with very little in common (bar being there in the first place).

It differed from my last theatre experience in December 2020 in the sense that we were coming out of a difficult period, rather than about to go into one. A sense of 'we're getting there, isn't this great!' rather than 'oh God, this is desperate, and even this will soon be taken away'. I left the theatre positive and full of hope.

Step Four – 'Freedom Day' – was scheduled for 21 June. Cases had begun to rise, and we had a new variant: Delta. As a result, international travel bans were brought in and Freedom Day was delayed until 19 July. But at least there was no reversal to Step Two, and I hoped and prayed the government would hold its nerve.

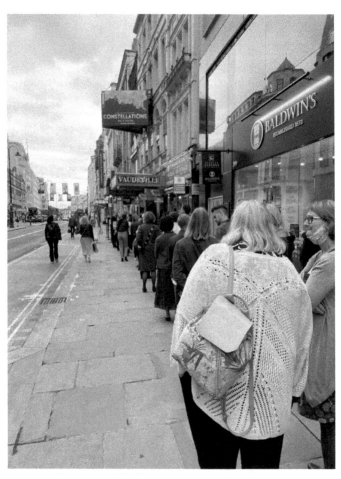

Queue for 'Constellations' starting Zoe Wanamaker and Peter Capaldi. June 24 2021

18 School's Out Forever

On one level July 2021 started extremely well. The City of London awarded me a large grant from their concessionary Covid fund. This fund had been set up to help businesses like mine that had fallen through the cracks of support. With this I received the same amount of support as businesses from other sectors. It was all I had asked for – this fairness in distribution. (I knew that whatever government policy was, people would have decided to work from home and companies would have closed their offices – my business would have suffered either way.) I was very, very grateful to those who pleaded my case and that of others, mostly my landlord and my MP.

Cases had continued to increase dramatically, as did the pressure to postpone or reverse the steps out of lockdown. But with the European Football Championship taking place early in the month, we seemed to skip Step Four and go straight to Step Five – a hyper socialisation if you like (not so dissimilar to my initial ski trip) with people mixing much more than they would do normally. When Freedom Day went ahead on 19 July (with the tournament over but schools yet to break up), it was followed by a collapse in the number of new cases; the curve seemed to have turned anyway, and its overshoot seemed more rapid due to the relative drop in football-related contacts.

In direct contrast to football, the last term of the school year had descended into farce. Any positive cases (more picked up as a result of twice-weekly testing) resulted in all close contacts having to isolate for ten days, even if their tests were negative. By the end of the term in mid-July, there were approximately one million children off school and isolating at home in the UK.

No school day could be taken for granted. My daughter's school had arranged a Year Six graduation with parents to try to gain some semblance of a rite of passage. It was to be held two days before the end of term with a party to follow and then a whole-school prizegiving to finish off on the last day.

The graduation was an odd affair. Masked, of course, we parents sat distanced from each other, another parallel experience rather than a shared one. It was important for the children, and I was glad they did it, but it lacked the crackle of camaraderie. There had been no shared experience between the parents or between the parents and the school. There was no school community.

Living so centrally there is always movement of children between schools, particularly between junior schools. In my daughter's year, about half the children had joined in Year Five or Year Six. Looking around the church where the graduation was held, I knew perhaps a third of the children and precious few of the parents. In my older daughter's year, I knew them all.

That evening at 10 pm we had an email from the school. One of the children in Year Six had tested positive on a lateral flow test, and the whole year had to isolate for ten days. There would be no class party the next day and no prizegiving the following day – the last morning of junior school. No head girl or head boy speech and no performance from the chamber choir – the first live one of the school year – on the last day. They would be isolating at home.

They were utterly, utterly miserable. Inconsolable. That the child's PCR result came back late the next day as negative and all the children were allowed to attend prizegiving (without an audience) was a relief, but the rollercoaster, yet again, meant they had to hold their breath. Not to relax, not to enjoy, not to trust.

Most of the children at my daughter's school were foreign nationals. They were not going to run the risk of having to stay in London under house arrest when they were due to leave for the summer, and some were due to leave forever. Some left that day, just in case.

Prizegiving went ahead. On video. We couldn't hear the head girl's speech or the head boy's speech. We couldn't hear the chamber choir singing. The tech had failed. Quite fitting, really. Far from being a celebration, the last two days of junior school became the latest disappointment in a long list of disappointments, and for me this chaos reflected how badly we, as a country, had let our children down.

My older child left junior school in July 2019. Her last year had been a period of change, a series of stepping stones to ease the transition. A maturity in forming and nurturing friendships, figuring out conflict resolution, how to work in a team, sports, music and debates. Step by step she had been allowed to grow.

There had been concerts, sports days, swimming galas and a school production. Prefects would walk the four-year-olds to the whole-school assembly every Tuesday morning. A school community. They had enjoyed a cultural week away at the beginning of the final term. Their end-of-year prizegiving had been an opportunity to celebrate and reminisce.

A consolidation of everything she had learned, educationally and emotionally, and an opportunity to say goodbye.

The Year Six party had been an outpouring of tears, emotion and resolutions to stay in touch. It had been a rough ride at times, particularly during the time of senior school exams and interviews, but it felt like they were well prepared for the change. The next time they would leave school would be as adults. This was the halfway point. Still emotionally immature but able to express and inform themselves and start figuring out who they were. With a strong emotional and academic foundation, and with the basics in place, they were ready to look out and discover the world and what their place would be within it.

My younger child, two years later, had a vastly different experience.

All rites of passage had been cancelled. They had been isolated from friends and peers continuously for almost a year and a half. When schools reopened in September 2020, there were bubbles, no mixing between years and no concerts. Parents were not allowed to enter the school, so they had little relationship with it. There were no performances, no sports fixtures and no school trips. No parties, no sleepovers and no visiting friends' houses.

And then in January 2021 schools closed again. This time it was the depths of winter. This time there was no optimism, only resignation. They slipped back into the routine of Lockdown One, hitting the emotional bottom within days, rather than weeks.

Instead of gaining maturity, they lost it. They were stiff, brittle shadows of their previous selves. They found it difficult to make eye contact. They would shuffle along hanging their heads with no swing in their arms, their faces blank, all sparkle gone. Not only had they been denied over a year of childhood development and experience, but they had also learned pain and loss.

Whilst some older children had the language to express their distress, the younger ones seemed to internalise it. Even when the opportunity to do something fun became available, they were no longer interested. With nothing to talk about, they didn't call their friends. They retreated further and further out of reach.

Some older children had broken down, shaking and sobbing uncontrollably after they finally returned to school. The younger ones just stayed missing. They checked out.

They couldn't imagine a time when this would be different. This was their normal. As children do, they lived in the moment and the recent past; all expectations of the future were determined by the restrictions of the pandemic. They couldn't remember the 'before' times.

I was tasked with making a yearbook for the end of the school year. For my older child this was a laborious but joyous and straightforward task. Each child had a page filled with images of their favourite school experiences. How on earth could I do this for Year Six part two?

I had to acknowledge the pandemic; it wouldn't be authentic without it. And there would be no pictures of school activities because they hadn't happened. I decided to write a questionnaire to put alongside one single favourite photograph. One of my questions was to ask them what they would do with all their masks once the pandemic was over. The answers were both illuminating and tragic.

> 'Throw in the bin, bye Covid.'
> 'Save them until the next pandemic.'
> 'Put them on my plushies or make a piece of clothing.'

'I will keep all my masks for future generations.'

'Draw on them.'

'I don't have any.'

'Build sails for miniature boats.'

'Keep them and still wear them because they match my style.'

'I will make a huge mask ball and throw it at someone.'

'Burn them and flush their ashes down the toilet.'

'I will sell them to get money.'

'I will throw them away and be overjoyed.'

'Burn them then make a wish.'

'Throw them away as quick as I can.'

To acknowledge the difficulties they'd had, I turned to Twitter for advice. What quotes could I use to acknowledge pain but be optimistic for the future? Here were the two I used:

> True happiness is to enjoy the present, without anxious dependence upon the future, not to amuse ourselves with either hopes or fears but to rest satisfied with what we have, which is sufficient, for he that is so, wants nothing.
>
> Lucius Annaeus Seneca (Thank you, Mary.)

> Keep your face always toward the sunshine - and shadows will fall behind you.
>
> *Walt Whitman* (Thank you, Elizabeth.)

And in a moment of self-indulgence, I added:

> This yearbook is not about academic, creative or sporting achievement. It is intended as a recognition of our children's values, their sense of humour and their resilience when many joyful features of their lives were taken from them. This is not a story about the pandemic and what they have lost. It is a story of everything they have gained and will take with them to the next adventure.

When returning to school after two highly abnormal years, they were not only two years older, but also expected to behave that way. They were expected to have the maturity and the mental and physical development of an older child. And keep progressing from that point on.

My indulgent screed above was a cry of hope, but we saw how damaged so many of them were. We hoped they would recover in time. We had to believe it. But for many this has yet to be undone, if it ever will.

No matter the age of your child, they missed an important, critical phase of their childhood. They will never get this back. They learned pain and loss at a formative time. Many lost their childhood, their joy and their rosy view of the world. Their uncomplicated seizing of the moment. And though I will try my hardest to forgive, I will never forget those who pushed to bring this about.

19 British Summertime

After school broke up for summer in July 2021, a school friend invited my daughter to perform at a street festival in Clapham outside her house. I had no idea what to expect but thought it would be a fun, relaxing and light-hearted affair, and nice for her that she had made some new friends.

It was a scorching hot day. My daughter had travelled earlier to rehearse, and the rest of us also travelled down a little early to have a drink in the sunshine. Walking up the steeply inclined street from Northcote Road, we were greeted by an array of plastic chairs arranged outside with several groups of parents and neighbours man-handling ice buckets stuffed with sparkling wine. It was immensely civilised and very British. But it didn't prepare me for what came next. My daughter's ensemble was a version of 'Comedy Tonight' on five different instruments. Many other solos, duets and trios too – a very high standard.

But one wee girl completely blew me away. Barefoot in a green floral jumpsuit, this ten-year-old girl gave the most astonishing performance I think I have ever seen, and I have been fortunate to see many. Huge, sweeping strokes of her bow, the emotion weeping from her violin as she delivered Fritz Kreisler's 'Praeludium and Allegro'. What this child with bare feet managed to convey, with the utmost poise, reminded me what raw emotion was. I had no idea how she had acquired the maturity to communicate joy and sorrow in such a powerful, searing way.

I sat and wept, swallowing down my tears, hiding behind my sunglasses. These children had been robbed of this, all of this, for eighteen months. It didn't matter what the source of your child's joy was, whether it was music, sports or simply playing with friends in person, it had been forbidden. They were expected to have reached the maturity of their chronological age without allowing the human socialisation necessary to achieve it.

All I read about was learning loss. What I cared about was life loss. That time as a child when you can laugh without hesitation, experiment and learn from your mistakes and those of others. Figure out who you are, how to relate to the world and your relationships with others. Whether that is learning to talk and interpret emotions from unmasked faces as a toddler or, when older, your first crush, your first kiss. Your first love.

For the school holiday we planned to stay in the UK since many countries had banned unvaccinated travellers, and vaccination hadn't been offered yet to the twelve-to-fifteen age group. So, we made the most of it and travelled around visiting friends and family for a week in Edinburgh for the fringe festival. Scotland, only five days before our trip, had announced a relaxation of restrictions, making it possible for shows to run. We had to wear masks, of course, and the chairs were separated and distanced, at least as much as possible in what were tiny venues. They all had electric fans too. This didn't seem to make sense: there were often no windows, so their only effect would be to circulate what was already there. They also made it much more difficult to hear what was happening on stage.

It was very quiet; the Royal Mile was deserted, but it picked up as the week went on. It rained almost constantly. The shows were, as expected, hit-and-miss. But it was a lot of fun to see the children laugh or squirm with embarrassment.

At the end of August my daughter was able to rehearse and perform with her youth orchestra. To see the children mingling, smiling and beaming with joy, both at the end of each day and during the performance, was such a relief.

For the end-of-course performance, social distancing reasons meant we were only allowed one ticket per performer. But despite sitting alone and having a parallel experience yet again, it was a step towards normality, and I was pathetically grateful for the experience.

The vaccination of children was a hot topic. The JCVI (Joint Commission for Vaccination and Immunisation), which decided who should be offered the vaccine, did not approve their general use in the twelve-to-fifteen age group, since costs and benefits were neutral for the children who were not particularly vulnerable. This was overturned by the government on the basis that more vaccinated children would mean fewer school isolations. We did not want to see the same debacle we had seen the previous term, and many parents were persuaded to agree to it specifically for that reason.

20 What To Do, What To Do, What To Do?

In September 2021 the City started to wake up. It started with the TWaTs (Tuesday, Wednesday and Thursday office attendees) – those who returned to work in the office on the middle days and continued to work from home on Monday and Friday. Appointments at my clinic jumped by 30% in the first week of September and continued to rise, albeit more slowly, from that point. I had to stand up on the tube for the first time since the beginning of the pandemic. Where 'business casual' had been normal attire, men in formal work suits and women wearing heels reappeared. Within two weeks Mondays and Fridays started to fill up too. I needed to recruit more staff.

But could I risk it? What would happen when Covid cases inevitably started to rise in the winter? Would the work-from-home trigger be pulled again? How on earth could I plan when I didn't know what the criteria would be? I had lost one-third of my staff due to the pandemic, and we were now at capacity. Campaigning for more restrictions had continued with a recent plea for another circuit-breaker lockdown to ease pressure on the NHS.

I wondered just how long people thought this waxing and waning of restrictions and lockdowns dependent on case rates could go on. Some seemed to think indefinitely. Our lives could be constantly on hold; no plans could or should be made that couldn't be cancelled at the last minute. No accumulation of harms would ever temper this demand when cases rose. How could it? This was now the standard protocol: when cases rise, we act.

What should I do? For my business, for my family, for me? I had no idea.

I decided to wait, just a little longer.

I read and read and read about childhood vaccination and still couldn't make up my mind. Research had been announced into the disruption of menstrual periods, and this was weighing heavily on my mind. My friends with boys were worried about myocarditis. The NHS vaccination service had not set a date for my daughter's school.

I decided to wait, just a little longer.

September felt like a fresh start. *A Normal Heart* at the National Theatre was the first play I'd seen with a cast of more than three people. It was pared down with some distancing and masks, but it felt like it was as intended, rather than adapted. It was a fabulous play, brilliantly staged, and wonderfully and compassionately performed. There was enough of an audience to make us feel we had experienced something together. And the bars were open. Odd how that makes a difference.

Chelsea Flower Show took place in September rather than the usual May. Despite not being terribly interested in flowers, I always enjoy it. People come to London from their country lives wearing Barbour waxed jackets and carrying shooting sticks to rest on intermittently between the artistic show gardens and the enormous pavilion of flowers. Sometimes I look at the audience rather than the plants: three generations of one family with identical chins or noses, all tilting their heads in the same manner to stare intently at whatever detail takes their fancy. Sophisticated Latin names effortlessly roll off their tongues, 'Is that a *Helleborus agapanthus* I see?'

It is brilliant. I am torn between admiring the extraordinary skill and knowledge needed to produce something I could never have the patience or talent to master and wondering just how some of the sculptures on sale could ever inspire an impulse buy. I am strangely comforted by the ubiquitous presence of the John Deere stand – a tractor maker who also sells enormous sit-on lawnmowers – whilst wondering if I would want the hassle of owning a patch of grass large enough to need one.

It was packed. Packed full of people older than me, cheek by jowl, peering over shoulders at the far fewer show gardens than in previous years. Only about 1% of people were wearing masks. The elderly people here were the vulnerable, those who government policy aimed to protect. Yet with cases still high, they clearly didn't want this protection. They had decided to live life to the full.

This was a common observation. Some of the groups, who had been most compelled to obey and who were most restricted by the Coronavirus Act, had returned to pre-pandemic activity, unmasked and tightly packed. Perhaps the vaccines had changed the risk calculus for them, but it made the continued campaigning for restrictions seem more unrealistic. Again, the plea came to 'save the NHS'. But was it our job now, as a nation, to protect the health service, rather than it protecting us?

Children returned to school for the new academic year. Finally, extracurricular clubs could run, and children were allowed to mix outside their classes and their year groups. Sports, music and simply hanging out with friends at lunch were now permitted too. There were no masks either, and what was previously a muffled half-communication resumed its full effect.

The Bond movie *No Time to Die* was finally released in cinemas. This release was originally due in March 2020, but it was delayed repeatedly when restrictions were reimposed. I thought we would know the pandemic was over when we were finally able to see it. It was a lot of fun taking our children. They huddled up together on the Curzon Cinema sofa, turning away from the kisses and gripped by the story – it is always more fun to take them with us than leave them at home. It was a wonderfully fun, shared experience. Although I'm not sure they'll ever forgive us for reassuring them repeatedly with the words 'Bond never dies', when this time, he did.

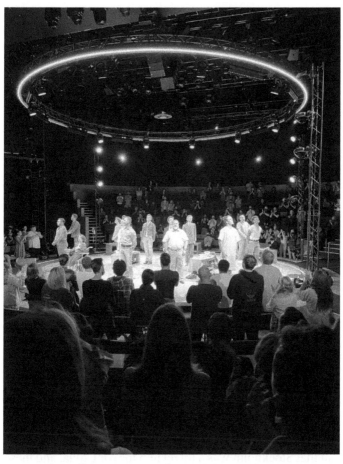

Curtain call for 'A Normal Heart' September 23 2021

21 A Very Different Capital City

The day after the cinema, on 3 October, one of my children woke up with a temperature. I didn't think much of it since the lateral flow test was negative, but I took her for a PCR test as per protocol. Two days before, we had booked a holiday for half-term and had started to get excited. Inevitably the PCR came back positive, and she had to isolate for ten days.

We couldn't go away. Although my daughter would be out of isolation, we were not allowed to enter this country if we had been in contact with her for two weeks after the isolation period had ended. She recovered quickly and was bouncing off the walls by the time she returned to school. We decided to go to Stockholm for a long weekend instead.

At Heathrow Terminal 5 we saw the astonishing sight of people in full hazmat suits getting on our flight. It turned out that Stockholm was a travel hub for Air China, and these travellers all peeled off to the transit queue after disembarking the plane in Stockholm.

Stockholm itself was a revelation. On exiting the airport we asked the taxi driver if he would like us to wear masks. He told us in excellent English (of course), 'No, we've done with that here. Coronavirus is finished in Sweden.' And so it would prove. On our touristy, busy weekend we saw maybe three or four masks in total.

Our weekend was a festival of meatballs, museums and clothes shopping. We enjoyed an exhibition of pet photography at the photography museum, with a glass of sparkling wine in our hands purchased from the unexpected champagne bar at the entrance to the exhibition. We visited the Abba Museum and the Vasa Museum. But my favourite memory of the weekend was of Skansen, the open-air museum park. This was reminiscent of London Zoo in terms of layout, but instead of monkeys and lemurs they had brown bears and gnus. We stood and watched the brown bears playing together for fifteen or twenty minutes before repairing to the food court. There you could buy sausages and marshmallows to grill on a large open barbecue, whilst you sat huddled up together on the benches that surround it.

Having visited London Zoo on many occasions when our children were younger, it felt very nostalgic: a reminder of a time when life was rather more straightforward. What I hadn't realised until then was how relaxing it was not to be confronted constantly by masked faces. Seeing them on our return to the UK was a reminder that all was not well. They put me on edge, not at ease. Of course, I understood that this was partly how they worked, as a visual cue to remind us to keep our distance from others. But after this incredible mental health holiday, to see them again made me recoil and flinch. It made me realise just how far we had to go on the route back to normal. And how much I had come to despise masks.

Yet there were many pleas for the return of masks and the return of working from home. Many had only just returned to the office. By the end of September, I felt sure many would be working from home again by Christmas. And that masks, however ineffective, would be bought back. I hoped I was wrong.

With the harms of lockdowns and restrictions better understood (due to routine data collection showing an increase in incidence of many conditions since the first lockdown), I imagined that a more nuanced strategy would be employed. Only use the restrictions that did reduce the rate of transmission, and only if these restrictions didn't cause more harm than good. I didn't understand why we would start to run the same experiment again without modifying the protocol to mitigate these harms. I'd foolishly imagined we'd keep the effective measures but abandon the ineffective ones in the hope that harms would be fewer.

The answer was still to have the option of using any or all of the restrictions, no matter how harmful, despite every adult having been offered a vaccination. Yet none of the adverse effects of masking or working from home were researched, plotted on a graph or considered as variables in a mathematical model. Our policymakers still seemed to be working blind.

The childhood vaccination programme had not stopped isolation in schools. They continued, along with masks, social distancing and reduced activities. They also changed the vaccination advice after infection. One day after my daughter had her first vaccination, and six weeks after she contracted Covid, the advice changed. Instead of six weeks between infection and vaccination, it was to be twelve weeks instead to avoid side effects.

Many parents were happy, enthusiastic even, in their consent for the Covid vaccination. But to have a situation where an eighteen-year-old A-level student would have to wear a mask and socially distance all day at school but could go straight to the pub afterwards to mix freely without a mask seemed nonsensical. It felt like our children had been held to a different standard from everyone else and for a much longer time, despite being the least vulnerable to the virus – consistently. After all, in the first wave the pubs reopened before the schools did, at least for the majority of children.

From the beginning we had been compelled to behave in a certain way for the greater good. This caused harms that we were not allowed to acknowledge or complain about. I'd complied with all guidance and mandates. I had contracted Covid in February 2020 and suffered Long Covid for six months afterwards. I had received my three jabs. I had volunteered for the NHS bank, had done some time on Test and Trace, had trained as a vaccinator and had worked at the Nightingale. I had nearly lost my business and accrued

£200,000 in losses. Those closest to me had suffered terribly.

I had already developed a strong dislike of masks. But in a post-vaccine world, and still with no robust real-world evidence to support their use, it became a hatred. I couldn't understand why, with such clear downsides and no strong evidence to show they worked in a community setting, they were still recommended. Masks came to represent my punishment at the hands of politicians, journalists and scientists. Because those people, in front of their screens and barely leaving their homes, would have to wear them much less often than others and they had been able to earn a living throughout whilst doing so. They wouldn't be the ones struggling to be heard, struggling to hear or suffering with 'maskne' (a skin reaction to the constant wearing of masks). It did not feel like we were all in this together.

The lack of acknowledgement that these protected lifestyles had only been possible because risk had been outsourced to others was disappointing. Essential workers of all types had been putting themselves at risk for the previous year and a half, the first year without being vaccinated. These 'same rules for all' meant that, whilst it was allowed for these workers to put themselves at risk in densely populated enclosed environments for work purposes, they were not allowed to sit on a park bench with a colleague after their shift. They couldn't even sit outside unless they had a garden. Which most did not.

Most people I knew who chose not to wear masks were those who had worked throughout. Had been exposed repeatedly. Were on the tube in May 2020 on the way to their essential jobs where they had no access to personal protective equipment. Or were changing at Canning Town tube station, massively overcrowded, in January 2021 during the third UK lockdown, before being offered a vaccination.

I couldn't understand those who were two vaccines in and still needed others to make them feel safe. And many privileged people who had worked from home were not vulnerable at all. On the other hand, many who were vulnerable, perhaps frail or at the end of life, wanted to see their families and hug their grandchildren.

Most people I knew didn't want restrictions to return. Most people I knew didn't want mandates or guidelines; they just wanted to be able to live freely. They wanted the old normal back.

It felt like we were never to be allowed to leave the pandemic behind. Our lives had already undergone a huge change, but some sought to make this change permanent. These restrictions, once established, were very difficult to unwind. The control of the public made governing easier and would be very difficult to relinquish. Why would those in authority have any incentive to relax them? We knew by then that the rules for our ruling classes were optional.

Masks came to represent everything I had lost and every pain I had suffered. I wasn't alone. The discussion around masks seemed to have been highly politicised, and this had only become more so.

To those who would have voluntarily restricted their lives in the absence of mandates, masks were a protection. To some of those working in healthcare, who saw many people die, they were a protection. Even if those people knew and acknowledged the lack of evidence, wearing a mask was a signal of comradeship, allegiance and respect towards those who had lost, suffered or been working on the front line.

But to so many others, masks came to represent their incarceration and their subjugation – the smothering of their needs and a visual confirmation of their irrelevance and unimportance. People felt dehumanised, with their only value being that of a cog in the machine, unworthy of individual consideration. Masking continued to separate us, both literally and metaphorically, from everyone else.

22 Under the Bell Jar

I have always loved to read. As a child I would hide my book and bedside lamp under a tent of sheets and blankets to prevent the light from leaking out around my bedroom door and giving me away. One time, sore from the contortion this required, I stuffed my dressing gown into the lampshade instead, dulling the light just enough to avoid discovery. It was only by chance that I didn't burn the house down: the scorched holes in my dressing gown were still gently smouldering in the morning when I eventually pulled it out, whilst investigating the curious smell emanating from the melting synthetic fabric.

I would devour three or four books per week. Thirsty for knowledge and hungry for experience, I tried to imbibe the wisdom that lay within as quickly as I possibly could. Now I read more slowly. I savour descriptions as much as plot twists, luxuriating in the complexity of language and the skill employed in delivering it.

I love real books, ones you can touch. Firstly, by visualising the cover I remember more about the book. I particularly love paperbacks, the more dog-eared the better. To me a previously read book is much more than the words and stories within: those words and stories contain a snapshot of my life. Perhaps the pages dried into corrugations after being dropped in the bath. Maybe some grains of sand were caught between the pages or a pressed flower that would tumble out on the next reading. Whilst the book leaves an impression on me, I also leave a physical impression on the book. When I reread, I remember what caused this sand, this water – and with it my thoughts and feelings at the time.

Mostly I read books to relax and escape. To immerse myself in the lives of others, fact or fiction. My interest has always been in how others see the world, the differences both inherent and conditioned. The human struggle. Reading allows me to process my difficulties in the same way as a night's sleep will provide the answer to a problem written down just before bedtime.

But since March 2020 I hadn't been able to read a single book. My consciousness was never silent; it buzzed with the task at hand or fretted over problems not within my power to resolve. I tried time and time again for the relaxation that reading would afford me. The tower of unread books on my nightstand remains a testament to my intentions and my failures.

But I was still living in black and white. A dulled half-life of drudge, routine and stress. My only ambition was to keep putting one foot in front of the other. Hoping, praying that one day it would be over.

It felt like a necessary strategy: to pace myself, drop a gear, and keep on going. Don't trust the odd peek through the curtain at my old, happy life. I knew that any freedoms may be short lived and could be taken away at a moment's notice.

I didn't feel great. I experienced huge swings in my energy levels. I still had brain fog, still felt anxious and still wasn't sleeping well. My body hurt. Repeated headaches, neck and back pain. I couldn't exercise the pain away because of the tiredness; my brain was too active to be able to sleep.

In addition to not being able to read, I'd stopped listening to music or participating in it. The constant, unremitting buzzing in my head drowned out any competing interests, even pleasurable ones. Outside my clinical work, I could focus for only five or ten minutes at a time.

I needed to do something about it. I was worried that the government might introduce a Plan B, as warned by the press, of masks and working from home, and I had nothing in the tank to deal with the fallout. I just needed to get through this winter, and I felt all would be more settled; at least I had to hope it would be.

I had no idea if these symptoms were menopause or Long Covid, and after a phone conversation with my GP, I booked an in-person appointment. She asked if I wouldn't mind having some medical students take my history. She would see me afterwards, but they could learn a lot from my story.

The morning of my appointment was one of 'those' days. One child was unwell, and I was worried; the other child was disorganised – a last-minute scramble. When I arrived to see the GP, I found that the morning was ringfenced as training time, and she wasn't allowed to see me for a consultation. I spent forty-five minutes talking to her students, then I went to work. When I got to work the internet was down, and none of our clinical notes were accessible. Quite a stressful start to the day, but by no means exceptionally so.

However, by the end of a full day of patients I felt completely spent. I had absolutely nothing left. I had no answers; I didn't know what to do next or how to approach the various things I had to deal with. The wheels had come off, and I ground to a complete stop. I sat on the tube going home and wept silently, grateful for once that I could reach for a mask to hide my embarrassment.

When I arrived to see the GP the following morning, she took one look at me and said, 'Mrs N, I've known you for years. You have been under an intolerable amount of pressure for an intolerable amount of time. You can't cope anymore. I can see it in your eyes, in the furrow of your brow. I call it the Dr M sign.' I was stunned. Even more so when she went on to flatter me, saying she had always admired how I had managed my practice (we had chatted about this often), juggling this with my children and family life. That she'd often thought, 'What would Mrs N do?' when dealing with a workplace issue. She went on, 'The thing I most admire about you is that you know when you cannot cope. You know when to ask for help.' My shock turned to immense gratitude. She had given me permission for my pain. I was not only allowed to admit my struggle but also applauded for seeking help.

It was OK; I was not a failure. Having spent the last twenty months under the impression that everyone thought my needs were selfish, unimportant and not a priority, someone understood. I had given everything I had. Again, and again and again. My vulnerability to restrictions was manifold, cumulative and unacknowledged by anyone in power, by anyone responsible for the decision to continue with them or to reimpose them. My GP prescribed me some antidepressants, advising me to stop these when the light started to return and the worst of the winter was over. She asked me to come back in ten days for the blood results (nothing remarkable as it turned out).

I had been completely unaware. Totally misdiagnosed myself once again. I thought my black-and-white life had been a necessary adaptation. It was not. It was the same disengagement I experienced when suffering from postnatal depression. What had surprised me then surprised me now.

You can't carry on being constantly numb. Your body needs to feel. So, it had given me mental and physical symptoms to try to get me to stop, take stock and allow some healing. But I hadn't listened; I was in no position to do anything about it. I couldn't stop being a mother, a wife, a daughter and a healthcare worker, or stop being responsible for my business and the livelihoods of those who worked within it. I had to keep going.

I realised my pandemic coping strategy was really a prison cell of depression and anxiety. Emotionally cut off, trapped within, suffocated. But unable to break out. Unable to breathe deeply. I'd continue like a wind-up toy: a spectator of life – not a participant.

Since February 2020 I had been trapped like a spider under a glass, which hadn't fully lifted to free me. To begin with I was a hive of activity, trying to find an exit, constantly on the go. Every time the side of the glass lifted, I would rush towards the gap and try to squeeze through. But by the time restrictions were lifted in July 2021, I was beaten. I would participate in the new freedoms; I thought I could fake it until I felt it. But I carried that glass with me everywhere.

No wonder I shut down. No wonder I dissociated from it. I walked around carrying this emotional burden for more than a year and a half, only allowing myself to stumble and fall when it was safe enough not to bring everyone else down with me.

Sylvia Plath's novel *The Bell Jar* describes a year of depression through the eyes of a young woman. It perfectly described the feeling of detachment I had endured with postnatal depression. It made a huge impact on me at the time, reading it during my recovery. Because for me depression wasn't sadness. I didn't sit and cry at home every night, feeling a loss of control over my life and my emotions. I felt nothing. I felt absolutely nothing. Dead on the outside, dead on the inside.

During the pandemic, bar the occasional fantasy of throwing myself off the nearest bridge, I didn't have full-blown panic attacks. I had learned how to cut these off, when to lie still, when to stare at the ceiling. Or touch and cuddle a loved one for the warmth of feeling that followed. This time I was a functional depressive, and I had a fabulous game face. I was getting through each day. Doing what was expected of me. I made it look good; I was convincing. Until I broke down completely on that journey home.

I had learned the error of my optimism. Even when the side of the bell jar lifted, I cowered in the corner. I couldn't see the sunlight anymore. Wouldn't see it anymore. Turned away, scared to believe, scared to let the rays heal my broken soul. I'd retreated so much that I had nowhere to go. So, I'd shut my eyes and wait for it to pass. Existing, not living.

I'd assumed my fatigue, muscle aches, pain, insomnia, anxiety and brain fog were caused either by Long Covid or menopause. But if I added my other symptoms of weight gain, pessimism, guilt, loss of pleasure, suicidal thoughts and restlessness, the dial shifted strongly towards anxiety or depression, or even both. After all these months of musing publicly on the possibility of a long pandemic – a generalised anxiety syndrome arising from pandemic stress and restrictions – I had missed it in myself. Fortunately, I had avoided the indoctrination of others, who may have thought my GP's opinion denied my physical symptoms.

Her diagnosis was right. It made me wonder if my self-diagnosis of Long Covid the first time had been in error too.

After two days on the pills, I had my first decent night of sleep in months. Over the following few days, the headache became more manageable, and I started to exercise. My pain began to settle.

The anxiety and brain fog would take longer, but I felt I had enough capacity to ride the winter wave of restrictions. I felt these were inevitable, whether justified or not.

23 Plan B: The 'Low-Cost' Cause of Long Covid?

On 30 November after the first two cases of the Omicron variant were identified in the UK, face masks once again became compulsory in shops and on public transport. Many international borders closed to travel, and anyone who had been in close contact with an Omicron case, vaccinated or not, was compelled by law to isolate for ten days. This was followed on 8 December by Plan B, which included the instruction to work from home. Two weeks after I had finally cracked and taken on a new member of staff, my numbers dropped by 30% and I stopped being able to pay myself once again.

This time there was a widespread backlash from the general public, taking many journalists, scientists and politicians by surprise. But with the long, slow release of lockdown, we were told there would be no backwards step. Going into winter, with people returning to their offices and school activities recommencing, it had felt like the last stage in the pathway to normality. Everyone was holding on. When Omicron came people cracked. With its arrival, all the pain and frustration of the pandemic came tumbling out.

Many hit the wall. I met so many people during that time, professionally and personally, who felt they couldn't go on. There had been no time to reflect, lick wounds or think about the future. They had been separated from their families, watched their loved ones suffer and hadn't been with them when they died. They had been banned from touching or having sex with anyone outside their household. They had miscarried alone. They were vaccinated, and more than 90% had antibodies. They had complied with restrictions for the greater good, without complaint, even when personally harmful. They had not been able to express their pain; they had to internalise it.

These are people who, like me, had hidden their distress from the people around them. People who, from the outside, you would never imagine were struggling. From my position treating patients for thirty minutes to an hour at a time, I was used to finding out how people were coping, or perhaps not coping. Functional, but miserable. So many taking medication to help them get through, just like me.

The reports that this new variant may break through previous vaccine and infection immunity made me feel that all this pain and sacrifice had been for nothing. We were right back at the start.

Of course, it was a disaster for office parties and hospitality. Nobody would risk being commanded to stay at home for Christmas and not see their families for the second time. So, all the end-of-year social parties were cancelled. There was no chance to let off steam and socialise with colleagues; many would have been doing so for the first time. People started working from home before they were asked, just in case. We all hoped this wasn't the first step back into lockdown.

We did, in the end, manage to spend Christmas with our families. But time and time again our lives had been restricted to protect others who may not have shared our vulnerabilities. It seemed to me that post-vaccine there was no longer any possible justification to inflict restriction harms. Pulling the rug from under people, even after the successful vaccine booster programme, felt cruel and pointless.

Some didn't see any issue with the working-from-home order, which was another 'low-cost' policy. But just like the assumption that in-person schooling could be adequately replaced by laptops and free broadband, the assumption that work and social contact online could be as successful, nurturing and productive as face-to-face contact had quickly broken down in a real-world environment. Before the first lockdown companies had made plans, with most of their staff working from home at least a week before the lockdown was announced. But whilst online video conferencing was useful for the dissemination of information or one-to-one collaboration, companies told me they had realised that collaboration and innovation simply didn't work as well online. Senior team leaders realised that their juniors needed mentorship.

Many of the juniors had struggled with lockdown. Some senior staff were overcompensating for their lack of presence by scheduling back-to-back Zoom calls, leaving the workers precious little time to do their actual work (or so the juniors told me). The juniors were expected to do this outside their paid working hours. I started to wonder if working from home was a significant driver for stress-related disorders and the same symptoms as Long Covid. Had this working-from-home order pushed them beyond their threshold for illness? Much as I had been fooled by my symptoms, how many others were misattributing theirs? How many of these symptoms had working from home in isolation with a huge workload caused in this group of people?

Working from home seems to work well when there is a need to focus on a specific task without interruption. Open-plan offices, originally designed to prevent siloed working, had made it very difficult for staff to concentrate on the task at hand. This had been discussed in occupational health circles for several years. But for collaboration, training and mentorship needs, in-person working is vastly superior. A hybrid solution separating these two job roles into work and home, with meetings at work and concentrated work from home, if possible, seems the best solution.

I investigated why video conferencing was so problematic and found some interesting opinions. The newly named 'Zoom burnout' was one opinion, leading to forgetfulness, difficulty concentrating, difficulty maintaining relationships, frustration with co-workers and physical symptoms such as muscle tension, pain, fatigue and insomnia. Another opinion piece hypothesised that Zoom headaches and fatigue arose from concentrating hard to make up for the lack of non-verbal communication.

What really intrigued me were the papers I read looking at the differences in the response between in-person meetings and virtual ones. These papers found that online social contact is only nurturing if you are connecting with those you already know well. If you are not, it increases stress rather than reducing it. This made sense. Coming off a conference call with someone you don't know often leaves people worrying about how they came across. Another interesting paper found that conducting an activity online makes you feel less emotionally connected to it. You are, after all, watching through a screen, watching a movie of your life, rather than living it.

We have known for some time how the brain and body respond to social media. Online attention causes a cortisol release, resulting in a neurochemical high and a compensatory low when it's gone. Are we sure that moving everything online, including most social contact, won't make us more stressed and anxious, rather than less?

The medical papers I read on the effects of social isolation were shocking. I read that it causes a plethora of symptoms and that the quantity and quality of social relationships are strong determinants of mortality. That the magnitude of the effect of social isolation is on a par with, and in many cases larger than, excessive drinking, smoking and obesity. Social isolation has been identified as a risk factor for violence against others. It is also of great relevance to mental illness, including social anxiety disorder, with a key feature being the avoidance of social situations. Those who socially isolate or withdraw have a more severe illness.

Considering all we know about the maintenance of mental and physical health, are we sure that encouraging online interaction over in-person interaction, including work, hasn't resulted in the very symptoms of Long Covid we were trying to avoid? Brain fog, muscle tension, pain, fatigue and insomnia? And anxiety? Barring joint pain, these are some of the most commonly reported symptoms of Long Covid.

24 Don't Worry, It *Is* Covid

On 19 January Boris Johnson announced that Plan B restrictions would end on 26 January. This time, despite my expectations, restrictions had not been the first step on the pathway to a full lockdown.

Since the build-up to the first lockdown, my butterfly brain had struggled to settle on anything, but within hours of this announcement my brain fog lifted. For the first time since the start of the pandemic, I could focus hard for more than five minutes at a time. The tight knot of nausea – my constant companion – slackened like the hair shaken free from a bun. My sleeping was once again unpunctuated by hourly glances at the clock. I would awake refreshed, not as lifeless as a rag doll.

My world finally returned to full, beautiful, breathtaking colour.

Walking through London's parks I smelled the green of early spring. The midday sun bleached away the vivid colours of winter. Narcissi emerged from the long grass, their top-heavy blooms swaying gently in unison, blown by the mild gusts of wind. Fewer ducks buried their beaks deep within their plumage.

In the City the arrival of spring allowed the sun to find pavements between closely stacked buildings, whereas in winter there was only darkness. Office workers, who had scurried from their office to tube station or sandwich shop, now sat or stood outside, inhaling this unique city petrichor through their unmasked noses.

Conversations moved on from distress, fear and loss to hope. Plans to visit distant loved ones. New restaurants, new plays. New friends, new lovers. More and more people tiptoed outside, regained confidence and started to remember and delight in this unfamiliar freedom. They'd carried the pandemic weight for so long they'd forgotten what it was like to live without it.

Work corridors became a burble of chatting, catch-ups and collaboration. Some returned reluctantly but were quickly inspired by the forgotten crackle of innovation and camaraderie of their in-person work environments. The most resolute of work-from-homers told me they felt excited about their work for the first time since the beginning of the pandemic. The City was alive again.

Tourists returned. Where we had been the only diners, restaurants now had queues around the block. Striding through empty Soho became once more a weaving manoeuvre through crowds of diverse fashions and different languages. Street performers returned, including the forgotten Yoda statues teetering precariously on their walking sticks, whilst appearing to float in the air.

My daughter and I had the opportunity to see *Tosca* at Covent Garden; the theatre was rammed to the rafters. A very, very special moment for us to share. Listening again to the piece she had learned in Lockdown Three ('E lucevan le stelle') caused us to weep silent, grateful tears behind our masks.

What an incredible feeling! I hadn't realised this step was still lacking. I also knew that, as with most Londoners, I would soon return to navigating my way through the back streets, becoming impatient with the random stuttering, stop–start walking pattern of those with time to kill. But for now I soaked up this atmosphere. London was back.

My fear became that lockdowns would be recorded only as a success with unfortunate, but unavoidable, collateral harms. The dialogue needed to start reflecting the reality that I had seen and that so many others (I believe the majority) had suffered. And I felt brave enough to start to look at my pandemic records.

We were lucky enough to go skiing again at half-term. Though I didn't feel lucky. I didn't want to go. Two years previously I had caught Covid in Austria, and all the pain of the pandemic began at that point: emotionally it was the start of the pandemic for me. But I was very lucky to be going skiing, and I didn't want to avoid it or have Covid lurking in my subconscious continuing to inflict its damage. The words of the psychologist 'don't avoid knives' rang in my ears. Build pathways around it, I thought. I didn't think the holiday would happen; after all, none of our trips booked more than three days in advance had happened for the last two years.

I actually hoped that one of us would test positive before we went. That I would have an excuse to sit back and take stock. The physical effort of packing and going away seemed too much. Until I admonished myself for my privilege, resolved not to be grumpy and decided to make the best of it.

The trip happened. Our PCR tests were all negative the day before, so we flew to France for half-term.

On Tuesday night I had a sore throat. On Wednesday morning it was worse, a lot worse. I tested myself. The T and C lines on the lateral flow device appeared almost simultaneously. I couldn't believe it.

The same Wednesday of February half-term, two years since my first Covid infection, I had Covid for the second time. On this occasion two of my family members also had it. Again, I was very unwell and quite glad the isolation allowed me to rest. Seven days in a ten-foot square room with my husband was an interesting experience, but at least the food was good.

I had been so grumpy about the prospect of skiing. We didn't stay in a self-catering apartment; we stayed in a hotel. With amazing food. Brought to our door by slightly bemused-looking waiters; our impression was that they couldn't believe we were bothering to self-isolate. I was delighted that, once again, Covid hadn't affected my taste or smell. It could have been a lot, lot worse.

Of course, when we came down to breakfast on our last morning in France we were surrounded by tables of coughing and spluttering fellow guests. It was clear that our willingness to test and isolate put us in the minority. Many people had ignored their symptoms and had no requirement to test if travelling from within France. I found this mildly irritating, but in one sense it brought me relief. If we had rebelled against the rules, maybe they wouldn't have been imposed on us for so long. If we had all done what we were told, would coronavirus restrictions ever have ended? These restrictions would make it easier to govern and police us, after all.

But I really couldn't believe it. At least this time I would be able to recuperate more and hopefully avoid Long Covid. In one way it was a fitting bookend to my pandemic story.

I called this chapter 'Don't Worry, It *Is* Covid' because at the time of the first infection I had a real reason to fear it. With three jabs and a prior infection, I no longer felt at risk of serious illness. (I was probably just as ill because I'd put on weight, had been very stressed and hadn't recovered my fitness.) Of course, I was still sensible. I had a SATs monitor to check blood oxygen saturation (this was before the research was published on its lack of usefulness), took plenty of rest and stayed hydrated.

But I never wanted to go skiing, ever again.

25 Epilogue: My Rules for Life

Observing my behaviour and that of others during these two years has been illuminating. With everyone a stakeholder during this pandemic, our human nature has been laid bare by the stripping away of politeness and magnanimity when we have all felt personally at risk, albeit for different reasons. We have shown others what we would usually choose to conceal.

There was no absolutist 'following the science' when the science was uncertain, so politics and bias had the casting vote. And with such a plethora of certainties from non-experts with grand-sounding titles, those with true subject expertise or those who acknowledged the need for trade-offs were hard to find.

Did online chatter and biased opinions in the national press and medical journals influence policy? I find it impossible to know. But it definitely influenced the information available to the public, and as such, I find it hard to imagine that it didn't influence public opinion. It surely informed our government which policies would be complied with and how successful they would be in trying to restrict our lives. Necessary, of course, for the purposes of compliance.

Whoever you are, bias borne of fear or personal risk is extremely difficult to override. Physical isolation from others seemed to steer many away from examining any negative effect of Covid policies on those least equipped to withstand them. None of those compelled to obey were asked if they wanted the protection of coronavirus restrictions. The only concern was to reduce transmissions, and since this would be the easiest to impose where people have the least agency, the rules were enforced most stringently on those with the least power.

We find comfort in unexpected places and at unexpected times. Many have been balanced and compassionate towards others whose circumstances they do not share. The milk of human kindness flows freely, but you may need to go outside your usual environment to find it. This compassion is not found within a tribe, whether political or financial, or in particular occupations. It has inspired me to seek out like-minded people who share my values, not my characteristics.

Calm heads make balanced assessments. Throughout this pandemic I have read and reread all the papers I had access to. But my most reliable opinions are shaped by the body of my prior knowledge. Nobody was without bias; we have all been stakeholders. But my prior beliefs, painstakingly refined and challenged when I did not feel at personal risk, have been those that have most held true. The lens of informed opinion, previously assimilated calmly and weighed dispassionately, has been my most honest witness. When I have been wrong, it was in areas where I had little prior knowledge, however deep a dive I attempted. I couldn't leave my personal circumstances out of my evaluation of new data.

Much of my specialist knowledge I assumed to be common knowledge. It is not.

It is my strongly held view that many people have forgotten how to be well. They don't understand that life without in-person human contact is unhealthy, and they campaign for 'vaccine plus' (restrictions to remain in a post-vaccine world), partly because they have become institutionalised by pandemic restrictions. Like Brooks in *The Shawshank Redemption*, they are fearful of the outside world. The incarceration in prison became Brooks' protection, with rules he could understand and comradeship that did not challenge. We should have compassion for people like Brooks. Those who contributed to their discomfort, not so much.

I may know some of my flaws, but I will never totally beat them. I may have silenced my inner critic professionally, but I still seek out the stimulus of information and push myself too hard. This is a fight I will never win. My excessive pursuit of knowledge and information was the symptom of not only my Covid anxiety but also my innate inner drive. Perhaps virtues and flaws are constant companions working in balance, like all human systems. I've come to believe you need to acknowledge and value both equally, as your flaws are what make and keep you human.

But none of us are exclusively virtuous. Worse, persuading yourself that your intentions are only ever honourable creates an opportunity for evil deeds. If you cannot question your motivations, you lack the insight to check your behaviour or to evaluate that of others. And the more power you hold, the greater responsibility you have to safeguard others from your worst instincts.

Learning something you find difficult can be extremely rewarding and fulfilling. It keeps you humble and gives you respect for others. Do things that don't matter for your work or self-esteem. Turn off your perfectionism. Draw badly. Sing out of tune. Give yourself permission to fail and keep failing.

I need to let go of the residual anger I have towards those who pushed for harmful policies. It will corrode me and have no effect on that which I despise.

I must remember to delight in the ordinary. Count my blessings because I have many more than most. We take too much for granted, but I feel lucky. Lucky that I find connecting with others to be quite so enriching. Lucky that I find pleasure in unexpectedly seeing a child learning to ride a bike, or hearing the gurgle of pleasure from a baby playing peek-a-boo. The sound of tidal waves when the wind streams through leaves in my favourite parks, or the cherry trees in full blossom. I just need to remember to be present in the moment, take time, take a deep breath and enjoy.

To move forwards my rules for life are simple. Get involved where you can make a positive change. Do not blindly trust the motivations of others, but always engage in good faith. Take time to look at the scenery, look up at the stars, not down at your feet. 'Know yourself', as Socrates put it. Find contentment in simple, non-expert pursuits. Live a life offline. Live a life more ordinary.

I move on from the pandemic better informed, poorer and scarred, but still able to appreciate what I hold most dear.

I am very lucky.

26 Reconciliation

Rereading the original draft of this book, I was taken aback by the anger within it. To direct my hate at individuals was perhaps my way to weather the storm, to fire up the mental energy I needed to get through and avoid complete collapse. Maybe it was easier to blame others than to take personal responsibility for the limited choices available to me, or perhaps it was simply a symptom of my clinical depression. Either way, I'm not proud of it. Reading it now, I am acutely aware of how little I have to complain about compared with others.

I hope that the information on health and wellness is informative, and perhaps that expressing my struggle will give others permission to acknowledge their own. For some it is best to move on without this type of reflection, as doing so will prolong the agony and worsen the harm. But for others, burying their suffering deep within can corrode from the inside and cause problems later on. Writing this book was partly a personal attempt to avoid the latter – to leave this book on the shelf and move forwards rather than carry the weight of it with me.

I often tell patients stories of my struggles to help them unlock their own. To show them it is normal to suffer and normal to question. Normal and human to make mistakes. This helps them gain some insight into how their mind and their bodily systems work together on a personal, individual level. It helps them identify what they have the power to change for an improved quality of life.

We need time to recuperate from the trauma of our pain and losses. And after this period of convalescence, to experience normal for long enough to trust it. To relax about it. To pick up the strands of forgotten parts of our lives and live our lives completely, without constant fear and apprehension.

Recovery is not constantly thinking about and evaluating your health: if you do that, you can often prolong symptoms by amplifying and reinforcing harmful pathways. Patients sometimes only realise they've recovered when it springs into their mind unprompted. Perhaps they get out of bed and remember how painful it used to be, then try to remember the last time they struggled to do it.

I imagine this will be similar for Covid. One June day in 2022, I left my home with a spring in my step, happy with the place I'd just left and happy to be travelling to my place of work. I reflected at the end of the day; there was a calm contentment to it, which was unusual. My old normal. Not the euphoria of a suddenly forgotten pleasure when something caught me off-guard. True happiness.

I realised then how much further I had to go. Of course, I had bad days before Covid, but these were made tolerable by the good and indifferent days around them. My good fortune in being able to relax, repair and renew gave me the strength to weather the inevitable storms of normal life. I also know that my recovery thus far has been possible because of my privilege. Many are not so lucky: they have buried their pain and loss, not having the opportunity to slow down, reflect and heal. The need to convalesce is not limited to physical injury, but whilst you can encase a fractured leg within a cast, there seems little recognition of the need to splint and support prolonged mental and emotional overload. It's no wonder there are high levels of sickness and widespread reports of burnout.

I hope that reading about my experience helps others to go through a similar process of catharsis.

For other people Covid won't be over for entirely different reasons. Some are still very scared of catching it. They have lived an isolated life for two years, and their world has contracted around them. Their normal has become a half-life; they accommodated it. Some even prefer it. I used to envy those who were able to isolate and still work; now I think they will take the longest time to recover and rediscover the beauty and necessity of human contact.

How can we move forwards? We have lived parallel lives. Due to the very nature of this threat and our imposed isolation, our experiences were not witnessed by others. We need to learn to live together again, to commune. To reconnect. To forgive.

We also need to feel heard. For others to acknowledge our losses. For those losses to be measured and considered.

Perhaps this is unrealistic. Will people be able to admit these harms? How important is it for us that they do?

I'm scared that restrictions will return. Terrified they are now the interventions of choice, with the full range of their knock-on effects uncollated and unevaluated in advance, during or afterwards. That the same voices will demand the sacrifices of others, time and time again. And that these voices will be heard by others similarly unharmed by these policies. But my belief is different.

I imagine that inflation and the cost-of-living crisis will end up being the barrier to the reimposition of lockdowns. I thought it would be the devastation that Covid restrictions caused, the human uncounted cost that would make them unpalatable but, cynically, I don't think this would be enough.

It should be to our collective shame that the poorest and most marginalised suffered the greatest from Covid, from the restrictions and now from the cost-of-living crisis – the latter caused in part by money spent on protecting others during the pandemic. These were our most vulnerable, always. And we failed to protect them. These individuals have lurched from crisis to crisis and to further crisis without power and without a voice. Whilst my good fortune has allowed me to recover, for them the harms have continued to accumulate.

Once the damage from the brutality of the criminalisation of human contact is fully understood and fully counted, I expect we will wonder how these mandated, policed restrictions could ever have been considered. Far from being a necessary evil, some of this damage, this devastating harm, cannot have been inevitable. I still fail to understand how it can be ethical to sacrifice our young for our old, or our least privileged for some of our most fortunate. Or how it can be morally justifiable to inflict harm on some to protect others against a risk they do not share.

Will we ever experience lockdowns again? I hope there's no need to consider them. I also hope that we never again take our good health for granted, and by doing so, destroy that which we hold most dear.

Most of all, I hope we have learned that good health should never be taken for granted. For if you remove what is required to maintain it, we are all, eventually, breakable.

Appendix I – Coronavirus Restrictions Timeline

12 March 2020

Anyone with new symptoms of a cough and high temperature is asked to isolate at home for seven days.

16 March 2020

Isolation with new symptoms is extended to fourteen days and extended to the whole household.

19 March 2020

Matt Hancock, Secretary of State for Health and Social Care, introduces the Coronavirus Act. This enables the government to restrict or prohibit public gatherings, control or suspend public transport, order businesses such as shops and restaurants to close, temporarily detain people suspected of Covid infection, suspend the operation of ports and airports, temporarily close educational institutions and childcare premises, enrol medical students and retired healthcare workers in the health services, relax regulations to ease the burden on healthcare services, and assume control of death management in particular local areas. The government states that these legal powers may be 'switched on and off' according to the medical advice it receives.

20 March 2020

Schools, pubs, restaurants, gyms and indoor leisure facilities are shut until further notice.

23 March 2020

The UK prime minister, Boris Johnson, announces the first three-week lockdown. People are told to stay home unless leaving for exercise (once a day), to buy food, seek medical attention or go to work (only when that work is legally permitted and cannot be done from home). Those who are extremely clinically vulnerable are advised to shield (not leave their homes unless for an emergency) for up to twelve weeks.

26 March 2020

Lockdown measures legally come into force.

16 April 2020

Lockdown is extended for three weeks.

11 May 2020

People are advised to stay two metres away from others and to wear face masks in enclosed public areas.

27 May 2020

The UK government launches the NHS Test and Trace contact tracing system.

1 June 2020

Outside retail businesses are allowed to reopen. Nurseries reopen. Some limited colleges and school years are allowed to reopen. Groups of six are permitted to meet if distanced and outside.

15 June 2020
All medical staff are to wear face masks. Non-essential retail opens with one-way systems, hand sanitiser, Perspex screens at tills and pinch points, and social distancing measures in place.

4 July 2020
'Super Saturday' – change of distancing to one metre plus (when two metres is not possible). Pubs, hairdressers, restaurants and tourist attractions reopen with risk-assessed, Covid-safe measures (social distancing, Perspex screens, sanitiser, temperature checks and one-way systems) and are asked to record names, contact details and arrival and departure times of visitors.

10 July 2020
People living in England are permitted to travel abroad to seventy-three countries without needing to self-isolate on return. The destinations are dubbed 'travel corridors' by the government.

24 July 2020
Face masks become obligatory in shops, supermarkets and on public transport.

23 August 2020
England's chief medical officer announces the opening of all schools with full Covid-safe measures including

bubbles. Children are only allowed to mix within their bubble, stay distanced within classrooms (including lunch) and take part in limited sports, music and extracurricular activities. Senior school pupils to wear masks.

14 September 2020
Rule of six: groups are limited to six inside and outside.

22 September 2020
Boris Johnson announces a 10 pm curfew and a return to working from home.

24 September 2020
Launch of the NHS Covid app. Users of the app are to scan a QR code to check in to leisure and hospitality venues. It is mandatory for hospitality, tourism and leisure venues, hairdressers and similar services, and local authority amenities to display a code.

14 October 2020
Start of the tier system of localised restrictions across England (London placed in Tier Two).

Tier One: Medium Alert – Covid-safe measures of masks, social distancing, hand hygiene, registration for contact tracing and Perspex screening plus:

- Rule of six indoors and outdoors
- Bars, pubs and restaurants to offer table service only: no orders after 10 pm
- Work from home if you can

- Education open with no contact outside bubbles
- Overnight stays of up to six people
- Avoid travel to Tier Three, only share a car with your household or support bubble
- Exercise indoors according to the rule of six
- Residential care: two people from a Tier One area with social distancing, no physical contact, PPE, hand hygiene, screens, visiting pods and window visits
- Large events limited to 50% capacity with all other Covid-safe measures in place
- Fifteen guests for weddings and wakes, thirty for funerals.

Tier Two: High Alert
- No mixing of households indoors, except for support bubbles
- Maximum of six outdoors
- Education, childcare and childcare bubbles permitted
- Overnight stays with household or support bubble only
- Avoid public transport and car travel with those outside your household
- Only essential travel to a Tier Three area
- Pubs and bars close unless operating as restaurants and serving a 'substantial meal' with last orders at 10 pm

- Fifteen guests for weddings and wakes, thirty for funerals
- No indoor exercise if any interaction with a different household
- Residential care: screens, visiting pods, window visits and outdoor/airtight visits only
- Work from home if you can
- Places of worship open, but no interaction between households
- Large events and sports limited to 50% capacity, or 2,000 outdoors or 1,000 indoors.

Tier Three: Very High Alert
- No mixing of households indoors or in most outside places except support bubbles
- Maximum of six in some public spaces, for example, parks and public gardens
- Education and childcare open
- No overnight stays other than household or support bubbles
- No travel outside area except for work or education, no car sharing or public transport
- Pubs, bars and restaurants closed, bar takeaway or delivery
- No group indoor leisure activities
- Fifteen guests for weddings and wakes, thirty for funerals, no wedding receptions
- Organised adult outdoor sports permitted, but only with household or support bubble

- Retail open
- Accommodation closed
- Indoor entertainment venues closed
- Residential care: screens, visiting pods, window visits and outdoor/airtight visits only
- Work from home
- Personal care open
- Worship open, no interaction between households
- No large events.

5 November 2020
Start of Lockdown Two. As Lockdown One, except education stays open.

2 December 2020
Second lockdown ends, return to tier system (London in Tier Two).

19 December 2020
The government announces a new Tier Four, which comes into force at midnight (mainly in London and the Southeast).

Tier Four: Stay at Home
- No household mixing except in support bubbles or two people meeting outside in public spaces
- Education open during term time, childcare permitted
- No overnight stays away from home

- No travel except for essential work or education, no travel into or out of Tier Four areas
- Bars, pubs and restaurants closed, bar delivery or drive through
- Indoor leisure closed
- Thirty guests for funerals, six guests for wakes, six guests for weddings in exceptional circumstances
- Exercise: allowed to leave home to exercise with your household or with one other person
- Non-essential retail must close from midnight
- Accommodation closed
- Entertainment closed
- Residential care: screens, visiting pods and window visits
- Work from home
- Personal care closed
- Places of worship open for private prayer
- Clinically extremely vulnerable to stay at home unless exercising or attending health appointments.

26 and 30 December 2020
More regions join Tier Four.

6 January 2021
Start of national Lockdown Three, including education closure.

15 February 2021
Start of hotel quarantine. The first passengers arrive at government-approved hotels as the travel quarantine

scheme begins in England. UK and Irish residents arriving in the country after visiting or passing through 'red list' countries must quarantine in a designated hotel room for ten days.

8 March 2021
Step One A of the roadmap. Schools reopen with restrictions. Exercise and recreation outdoors with household or one other person from a different household. Funerals permitted thirty attendees, weddings and wakes permitted six attendees maximum.

29 March 2021
Step One B of the roadmap. Organised outdoor sports. Maximum fifteen people meeting outside.

12 April 2021
Step Two of the roadmap. Rule of six or two households outdoors. Retail, personal care, libraries and community centres open. Indoor leisure opens, including gyms. Outdoor hospitality opens. Domestic overnight stays (household only).

17 May 2021
Move to Step Three of the roadmap. Maximum thirty people to meet outdoors. Rule of six or two households indoors. Indoor hospitality, entertainment and attractions reopen. Organised indoor sports reopen. All accommodation reopens. Domestic overnight stays out of household. Launch of the NHS Covid pass to show

vaccination status and gain access to international travel and leisure/entertainment.

19 July 2021
'Freedom Day' – the final step out of lockdown. Step Four: no legal limit on social contact. Remaining businesses open, including nightclubs. High-risk venues such as nightclubs, theatres and large group events encouraged to use vaccine passports. International travel permitted. No legal limit on life events.

27 November 2021
Face coverings become compulsory in shops and on public transport.

8 December 2021
Government announces Plan B – masks, mandatory Covid vaccine passes, work from home, fourteen-day isolation with a positive test.

26 January 2022
End of Plan B and all government-imposed restrictions.

25 March 2022
The Coronavirus Act expires.

Acknowledgements

There were many people who helped me in a personal or professional capacity throughout the pandemic. Workwise I was lucky enough to have the support of Becky, Jane, my MP Nickie Aiken, my patients (particularly when negotiating with insurers) and my amazing team at work, especially my fabulous secretary and dear friend, Ros Summers.

My Twitter support group, many of whom I've had the privilege of meeting in real life and am chuffed to now call my friends. You are too many to mention, but I'd particularly like to shout out to Mike, Amy, Rob, James, Thomas, Sunil, Michael, Georgia, Rachel, August, Clare, Ellen, Gemma and Lucy.

Those who were kind enough to support my writing, read my drafts and give useful feedback. Anna Maria, Faye, Jackie, Ben, Liz and Tom – thank you. And thank you to Tom Whipple for meeting me in person and giving me advice on how to publish my book, to Laura Dodsworth, who introduced me to a publisher, and to Liz Cole, who sent me some very helpful tips. I'd also like to thank Christopher Matthews and Tom Jesson for very useful Zoom meetings on self-publishing, and Louise Glynne-Walton for her editorial support.

A huge shout-out has to go to Robert Dingwall, who has advised me throughout, given notes on several of my drafts and written my foreword. You have been extraordinarily kind and patient with this first-timer; I feel extremely blessed to have had such support.

Finally, of course, my dear family. I love and cherish you, and I look forward, finally, to our next chapter.

Ingram Content Group UK Ltd.
Milton Keynes UK
UKHW021959220523
422165UK00013B/225